men's hairdressing

traditional and modern barbering

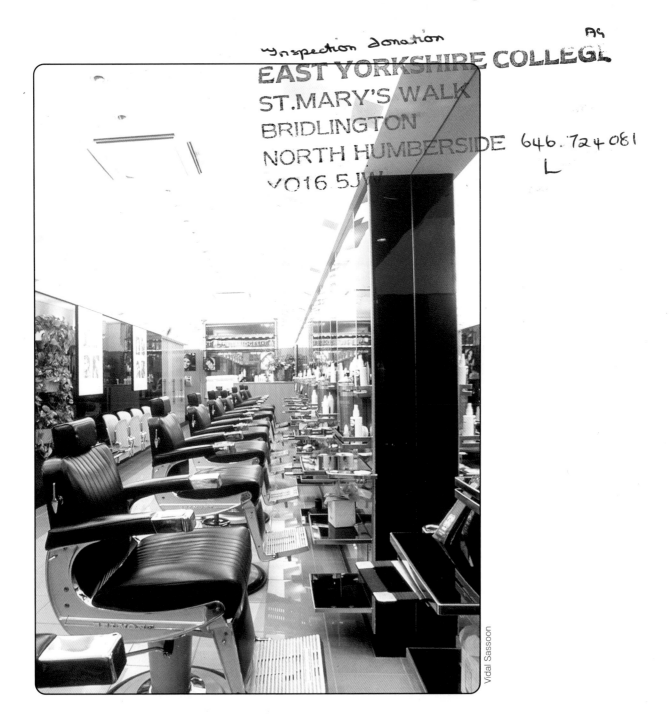

Vidal Sassoon

men's hairdressing

traditional and modern barbering

Maurice Lister

First published 2000 by
MACMILLAN PRESS LTD
Houndmills, Basingstoke, Hampshire RG21 6XS
and London
Companies and representatives throughout the world.

ISBN 0–333–73287–1 paperback

A catalogue record for this book is available from the British Library.

This book is printed on paper suitable for recycling and made from
fully managed and sustained forest sources.

10   9   8   7   6   5   4   3   2   1
09 08 07 06 05 04 03 02 01 00

Printed in Hong Kong

contents

EAST YORKSHIRE COLLEGE
ST.MARY'S WALK
BRIDLINGTON
NORTH HUMBERSIDE
VO16 5JW

acknowledgements   vi

foreword   vii

introduction   viii

■ 1 barbering – from its origins to the
      present day   1
      the origins of barbering   2
      barbering today   4

■ 2 client care for men   6
      client care for men   7
      consultation   7
      caring for your client   8
      preparing the client   9
      after-care advice   9
      the structure of the hair and skin   10
      the hair   10
      the skin   13
      the structure of the skin   14
      conditions of the hair and skin   16
      health and safety   20

■ 3 cutting facial hair   22
      cutting and styling facial hair   23
      consultation prior to cutting facial hair   24
      tools and equipment   26
      preparation for cutting facial hair   26
      cutting techniques   27
      a cutting procedure   28
      health and safety   31

■ 4 cutting men's hair   32
      cutting and styling men's hair   33
      consultation prior to cutting men's hair   38
      tools and equipment   44
      preparation for cutting hair   47
      cutting techniques   47
      cutting procedures   54
      health and safety   68

■ 5 shaving   71
      the professional shave   72
      shaving   73
      consultation prior to shaving   73
      preparation for shaving   75
      shaving materials, products, tools and
         equipment   76

      preparing razors for use   79
      preparing the beard   82
      shaving techniques   85
      a shaving procedure   86
      health and safety   90

■ 6 face massage   93
      face massage – effects and benefits   94
      anatomy of the face and neck   95
      consultation prior to face massage   98
      products, tools and equipment   99
      preparation for face massage   100
      preparing the face for massage   100
      face massage techniques   101
      a face massage routine   104
      health and safety   108

■ 7 drying and finishing men's hair   109
      the theory of blow-drying   110
      consultation prior to blow-drying   110
      preparation for blow-drying   111
      products, tools and equipment   111
      blow-drying techniques   114
      blow-drying   114
      blow-waving   116
      other techniques   119
      finishing techniques   121
      health and safety   121

■ 8 perming men's hair   122
      the basic principles of perming
         and neutralising   123
      consultation for perming men's hair   125
      perming in men's hairdressing   126
      health and safety   128

■ 9 colouring men's hair   129
      the basic principles of colouring   130
      hair colourants   132
      bleaching   135
      consultation for colouring men's hair   136
      colouring in men's hairdressing   137
      health and safety   142

index   143

acknowledgements

On a personal note, I would like to thank my wife, Dawn Lister, Suzannah Tipple, Andrew Nash and Isobel Munday at the publisher, and all at the Hairdressing Training Board, for their patience, encouragement and support, without which this book would still be just an idea.

The author and publishers would like to thank the following for providing pictures for the book: American Crew, Barrie Carter, Carl Shaw, Charles Worthington, Charlie Miller, Clinique, Comby, Daniel Hill, David Adams, Denman, Depilex/RVB, Dr Andrew L. Wright (Consultant Dermatologist, Bradford Royal Infirmary), Dr John Gray (Procter & Gamble), Dr Michael H. Beck (Consultant Dermatologist, Salford Royal Hospitals NHS Trust), Ellisons, EXIT Hairdressing, Goldwell, Hairdresser's Journal International, Hairdressing Training Board, JFK Edinburgh for Goldwell, John J. Dibbens for Staffords, Justine for Charles Worthington, Lee Stafford, Mahogany/Denman, Martin Turner/S.F.T.W. Barbers Shop, MK Hair Studio, Nigel Sillis, Olymp, Patricia Livingston/Renbow International, Patrick Cameron, Paul Stafford, Ralph Kleeli, Redken, Regis, Rita Rusk for Goldwell, Schwarzkopf, Carl Shaw, Simon Shaw/WAHL, S. Lewis, Sorisa, Thrive, TRESemmé, Vidal Sassoon, WAHL, Wella Great Britain, Wilkinson Sword.

The author and publishers would also like to thank the following: Simon Shaw, his colleagues and family who were involved in some of the various techniques photographs taken for this book, Sheffield College for the loan of a barber's chair, Ian Lea Photography for involvment in many of the step-by-steps which appear in chapters 3, 4, 5, 6 and 7. Special thanks to Barrie Carter for the offer of a photograph of his grandfather's barber's shop and to Nigel Sillis for supplying photographs of his father, Henry Sillis's barber's shop. Finally, thanks to all those kind people who have allowed us to use photographs of their hair.

foreword

In 1989 I joined the Hairdressing Training Board. One of the first things I found out was that men's hairdressing was in decline and that action was required to make sure that essential skills in barbering were not lost. We made the commitment to develop men's hairdressing and work hard to protect these special skills so that the future would be secure.

This book was produced in 1999. In the years since we made that commitment, the HTB has influenced the development of men's hairdressing by developing new standards and by running stimulating workshops. The result is a reversal in the decline of men's hairdressing.

And now, with the addition of men's grooming, men's hairdressing has become a distinct and acceptable section of the industry, with a secure future. I believe this excellent book will serve to develop the rich vein of talent that exists in UK hairdressing.

Alan Goldsbro
Chief Executive, Haidressing Training Board

Vidal Sassoon

introduction

Although men make up about 50 per cent of the population, traditionally few hairdressers have specialised in the barbering skills required to develop the men's business. Indeed, some traditional barbering skills were in danger of being lost. Recently, increasing interest in male grooming has provided additional business opportunities for the skilled barber and has, along with the frequent use of barbering techniques in women's hairdressing, further increased the demand for barbering skills.

I have written this book both to help address this demand and to help ensure that the traditional skills are not lost. Whether you are an experienced hairdresser or just starting out on your career, the book provides you with all the information necessary to help you develop your potential in barbering. For experienced barbers, I have also included information to help you consolidate your knowledge and skills, which I hope will in turn provide inspiration to develop new services and increase the men's business.

I hope you enjoy reading the book as much as I have enjoyed writing it!

Maurice Lister

Vidal Sassoon

1 barbering – from its origins to the present day

Nigel Sillis

Nigel Sillis

Vidal Sassoon

Barbering has a long and varied past which should be considered by anyone who has an interest in the work of the barber.

This chapter discusses the evolution of barbering to the present day and covers the following topics:

- the origins of barbering
- the meaning of the word 'barber'
- barbering in the ancient world
- the significance of 'barber-surgeons'
- the origin and meaning of the barber's pole
- the development of barbering techniques to the present day.

the origins of barbering

Barbering may accurately be described as one of the oldest professions in the world. Archaeologists have found simple cutting implements made from sharpened flints and bones, which show that haircutting was practised as long ago as 30,000 years BC. The Egyptians were the first to develop techniques and tools that we might recognise in hairdressing today. Excavation of Egyptian pyramids has unearthed many combs and cutting tools, including razors made of tempered copper and bronze that were used by Egyptians nearly 6000 years ago.

The word 'barber' derives from the Latin word *barba*, meaning 'beard'. Many barbering skills developed because of the importance of the beard in past times. A beard was often considered to be a sign of wisdom and strength and, not surprisingly, also of manhood. The beard has been important in many religions throughout the ages and in some is still important today.

barbering in ancient times

Organised **barbering services** were offered as long ago as 1500 BC. In ancient Egypt many men had their beard and their head shaved. Egyptian barbers often preferred to work outdoors, because of the hot climate. The barber would meet his clients in the street, where the client would kneel while the barber casually went about his work in full view of passers by.

Although popular in ancient Egypt, shaving did not become commonplace in most other countries until around 400 BC, by which time hairstyling and barbering had evolved into highly developed crafts.

In ancient Greece wealthy men regularly had their hair cut and styled, often by their servants, but most members of the poorer classes still wore long hair and beards. In about 335 BC Alexander the Great, ruler of Greece at the time, promoted widespread shaving when he ordered his army to remove their beards. This was a strategy to overcome his enemies' tactic of grasping the Greek soldiers' beards during battle. Alexander himself was clean-shaven, which was unusual at that time, when most rulers wore beards, and this too encouraged shaving as men who admired him copied his example.

Alexander the Great

In Rome by about 300 BC barbering services had become available to the general population. Slaves were still forced to wear their beards and hair long, as a sign of their lower status, but most other men visited the **barber's shop**. Roman men were usually clean-shaven so the barbers' shops were much frequented. They were used as meeting places, and were known to be good places to catch up with the local gossip. Many Roman barbers enjoyed considerable wealth and status in Roman society because of the success of these early shops.

barber-surgeons

By the Middle Ages barbering services were well established in England and across most of Europe, but barbers were no longer only shaving and haircutting. These early barbers were also the pioneers of many medical treatments. Because they performed both barbering and surgery, they were known as **barber-surgeons**. They frequently carried out bloodletting and simple surgery, and also pulled teeth – a simple form of dentistry.

bloodletting

the barber's pole

The familiar red-and-white striped **barber's pole** originated as the symbol of the barber-surgeons and their work in bloodletting. Bloodletting involved cutting a vein on the patient's arm, in order to let out 'bad blood'. Many ailments were thought to be caused by 'bad blood', which was sometimes said to have been affected by evil spirits. Although it was widely believed that removing this blood would bring about a speedy recovery, this treatment is not known to have been successful. On the contrary, infection would often develop at the site of the cut and this would lead to other serious illnesses.

Wounds were dressed with cloth bandages. In those days the bandages were used over and over again: although they were white at first, with repeated use they became stained. Whilst hanging outside the barbers' shop to dry, they would twist together with new white bandages, forming the red-and-white striped pattern familiar to us now as the barber's pole.

a barber's pole

Some barbers' poles also have a blue stripe, and a small bowl hanging beneath. In this instance the pole is said to represent the post that the patient held onto whilst undergoing treatment. The blue stripe represents the blood from the veins, the red stripe the blood from the arteries. The arteries should not have been cut at all, but sometimes they were, by mistake; this illustrates how hazardous the treatment was. The bowl hanging beneath is often said to represent the bowl used to collect the patient's blood. In reality, it is more likely to have been the bowl used to collect lather during shaving.

During the 13th century the 'Barbers Company of London' was established, to help regulate and protect the developing barbering profession. Within a few years some of the barber-surgeons began to favour surgery and formed a 'Surgeons' Company' or 'Guild'. In the middle of the 1500s, after many years of disagreement, Henry VIII of England created an Act that united barbers and surgeons under one corporation. Under this Act barbers were prohibited from performing surgery, although they could continue bloodletting and teeth pulling; and the surgeons were prohibited from performing barbering and shaving services.

The barber and surgeon had been united in one profession for over 500 years when they were finally separated in 1745. George II of England passed an Act that divided barbers and surgeons into two distinct corporations. The 'Worshipful Company of Barbers' was formed and barbers dropped their use of the name 'barber-surgeons'. Since then barbers have not performed any medical services, but in many high streets today you will still see the red-and-white striped pole as a symbol of barbers' long, varied and significant past.

■ barbering today

a modern barber's shop

Today the term **barbering** is usually used to describe the work carried out by men's hairdressers, gents' hairdressers, and men's hair stylists – all of whom might be described more simply as 'barbers'.

Regis

Vidal Sassoon

Vidal Sassoon

Of necessity there are many similarities between the work of men's hairdressers and women's hairdressers, but differences do remain between the work each carries out and by their use of different techniques. At one time it was very fashionable to have **unisex salons**, where both men and women could have their hair cut and styled. Unisex salons used barbering techniques but often did not specialise in **men's hairdressing**. A barber is someone who specialises in men's hairdressing, and who has developed high-level skills in using barbering techniques, especially for haircutting. These techniques are particularly suitable for dealing with men's hair and for creating men's hairstyles and beard and moustache shapes.

More recently, interest in male grooming has increased, as can be seen from the number of hair and skin-care products now available that are produced specifically for men. Many more men are wearing fashion haircuts and there has been a marked increase in the popularity of beards and moustaches, particularly with young men. This interest has led to many more barbers' shops opening and to an increase in the different services available to men. Today the barber has to be highly skilled and creative in most aspects of hairdressing if he is to meet the needs of his clients and create the varied range of styles that are required. As will become evident through this book, modern men's hairdressing is not just about a 'dry trim' or a 'short back and sides'!

Vidal Sassoon

Vidal Sassoon

2

client care for men

Client care is an essential part of any hairdressing service: it forms an important part of all barbers' work. Providing care involves you working to meet your clients' needs, so that they are satisfied with every aspect of the service you offer. Good client care is a sign of professional standards of work, which all clients should be able to expect.

Client care is achieved through many different skills, including good communication, technical ability, and good manners. The following are some of the important topics covered in this chapter:

- communicating with your client
- recognising the needs of your client
- preparing your client for different services
- caring for your client
- offering after-care advice
- knowing about the hair and the skin
- identifying hair and skin conditions and disorders
- determining when services should or should not be carried out
- salon hygiene.

client care for men

In essence, client care is the process of caring for your client, and it is the same for both men and women. It involves you looking after your client, ensuring that he is comfortable and safe throughout the service, and that ultimately he is satisfied with the end result.

Client care should begin when the client makes his appointment, which may be in person or over the telephone. It resumes when he enters the salon, and continues until he leaves. Client care should also feature in the offer of after-care advice. This involves you providing advice on after-care products and tips on grooming and styling to help the client maintain his style at home.

In the salon, the first, and essential, stage of client care is the consultation. This must take place before any service is carried out, both for new and existing clients.

Vidal Sassoon

consultation

Consultation is a two-way process between you and your client, whereby you identify the client's wishes, determine his suitability for the requested service, and provide advice on the most suitable course of action. It involves you both talking to the client and listening to him, so that you can accurately establish his needs. You will need to exchange ideas, and you may need to refer to photographs or sketches to help you clarify the ideas and reach an agreement.

tip

- Sometimes your client may have no idea of what he wants – you will need to use your professional knowledge to guide him. This is an opportunity to develop a good relationship and to establish a loyal client!

a consultation is *always* necessary

In the barber's shop clients sometimes have their hair cut dry. Indeed, you have probably heard the request 'A dry trim, please' on many occasions. It may seem as if consultation is unnecessary for such clients, especially if they are regular customers at your salon.

However, you must *always* carry out a consultation. This is an opportunity for you to find out about any problems the client has had with his hair which you could help correct. But more importantly, it is vital that you identify any possible infections or infestations, so that you can protect your other clients, your colleagues, and yourself.

talking with the client

Listen carefully to what your client says – after all, most clients usually know a lot about their own hair. Sometimes you may realise that a satisfactory result would not be likely: you will then need to advise your client to have a different service or a different style from the one he has requested. Remember to do this tactfully, and explain in simple and clear language the reasons for your recommendation.

As part of the consultation, you will need to examine the hair and scalp. The hair should always be *dry* when you do this, so that you can see any problems clearly. Proceed with the service only when you have accurately established what is to be done and have obtained the client's understanding and agreement.

Here are some important points to remember about consultation:

- be tactful
- observe the client's confidentiality at all times
- accurately determine the client's wishes, both before and during the service
- use your skills of questioning and observation to gather all available information
- where necessary, perform tests to determine what services can be carried out: ensure throughout that you work safely and protect the client from harm
- ensure that you identify any adverse conditions of the hair or skin – if you suspect that an infection or infestation is present, you must not carry out the service
- before proceeding, ensure that the client understands and agrees with the service
- take into account any hairpieces that the client may be wearing – determine how these may affect the services to be provided
- record information about the client accurately, so that you can retrieve and review it easily on his subsequent visits to the salon

tip

- **Never** carry out a hairdressing service without a consultation. It is unprofessional and is likely to result in a dissatisfied client, or worse!

■ caring for your client

Throughout the service, you must take care of your client and ensure that he is comfortable. This can be achieved by following some simple rules:

- **security** Ensure that the client's coat and belongings are placed safely in the appropriate place.
- **preparation** Gather together all the materials, products, tools and equipment you will require before you begin work.
- **comfort** Ensure that the protective gown, the cutting collar, towels, cottonwool pads and so on all remain in their correct places before and during services. During cutting services, remove excess hair cuttings from the client and the gown or cutting collar.
- **reading and refreshments** In accordance with your salon's policy, offer the client reading materials or refreshments, especially during lengthy processes such as colouring and perming.
- **explanation** As the service progresses, let the client know what you are doing – especially during perming, colouring or lightening. Explain how long the service might take, ask the client if he has any questions, and reassure him if necessary.
- **finishing** Ensure that the client's clothes are not damp or stained, and that all loose hair clippings have been removed. Return the client's coat and belongings to him. Offer to make the next appointment for him.

tip

- Make sure you make a record of any staining or damage to the client's clothes and inform your manager or supervisor.

preparing the client

gowning and protecting the client

Following the consultation, and before you proceed with the services to be carried out, the client must be correctly gowned and protected. Which gowns, towels and so on are needed will depend on the service to be performed: this is explained in more detail in the relevant chapters. Here are some *general* rules to follow when gowning and protecting clients.

- **the chair** Before seating the client, check that the chair is clean: remove any hairs that may have fallen on the seat or the back of the chair. Position the chair and the client in the correct position for the service to be carried out.
- **the gown** Place a *tissue* or *neck strip* around the client's collar, then secure a clean gown into position.

- **shampoos** If the client is to be shampooed, one or two towels will be required. For a *back-wash basin*, one towel should be placed over the back and shoulders. For a *front-wash basin*, one towel should be placed across his chest and tucked in at the neck, and a second towel placed over the shoulders and the first towel.
- **cutting** If cutting, use a **cutting collar** and/or **cutting cape**. Make sure no hair can fall down between the client and the chair back.
- **shaving** When shaving, place a clean towel around the front of the client. A **paper towel** should then be placed over the towel and across the client's shoulder (from his neck towards your body).

preparing the client's hair

The client's hair must be freed from any tangles before you can work with it effectively.

1 Begin by teasing the hair apart with your fingers. If the hair is long and very tangled, follow these simple steps.

2 Using a wide-toothed comb and beginning near the nape, take a section of hair and comb through the ends, removing any tangles. Gradually work up the section of hair until the comb will travel easily from the roots to the ends.

3 Continue taking sections in this way, working up the back and sides, until all the tangles are removed. Take care not to jerk the client's head whilst combing the hair.

after-care advice

You should provide advice on after-care products, and tips on grooming and styling to help your client maintain his hair at home. This is also an opportunity for you to suggest other beneficial salon services.

Here are some suggestions for you to consider:

- always offer advice and tips on styling to clients who have had new styles
- encourage clients to ask about services
- suggest products that will benefit clients most and keep their hair in good condition.

■ the structure of the hair and skin

Anyone with an interest in providing hairdressing services must understand the basic properties of the hair and the skin, and the effects that certain services have on their structures. The location and function of the *cuticles*, *cortex*, *hair follicles* and *blood supply* must all be understood, as these often affect the choice of techniques and how they are applied. The different *types of hair*, the *hair-growth cycle* and the hair's *chemical composition* and *physical properties* should also be known.

■ the hair

Hairs are to be found covering all parts of the body, except for the palms of the hands, the soles of the feet and the eyelids.

types of hair

There are three different types of hair.

lanugo hair

Lanugo hair is a very fine downy hair that covers the body of unborn and newborn babies. It is usually lost either at birth or soon afterwards.

vellus hair

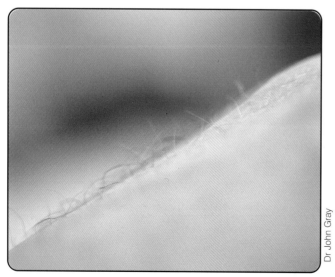

vellus hair

Vellus hair is very fine hair which occurs on most parts of the body. It can often be seen on the cheeks of women, and on the forehead and scalp of men with **male-pattern alopecia** (**baldness**), as the vellus hair is not usually lost.

terminal hair

Terminal hair is the longer hair that occurs on the head, arms, legs, eyebrows and pubic areas, and on the face and chest in men.

hair structure

Each individual hair shaft consists of three layers.

the cuticle

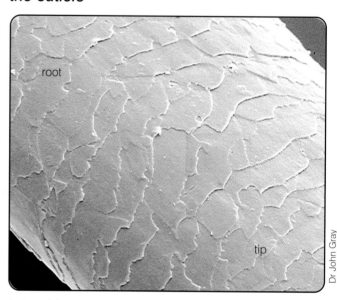

hair cuticles, seen under an electron microscope

The **cuticle** is the thin outer layer of the hair, which is made up of colourless **cells**. The cells look like scales and overlap like tiles on a roof. The scales point *away* from the roots and *towards* the ends: the hair feels smooth if you rub your hand from the roots to the ends, but rough if you rub it from ends to the roots, especially if the cuticles are damaged.

The cuticle forms a protective surface to the hair and so helps to maintain its condition. Healthy hair shines because all the cuticle cells are lying flat and the light is reflected. Damaged and rough cuticles trap the light, making the hair appear dull and lifeless.

the cortex

the hair structure

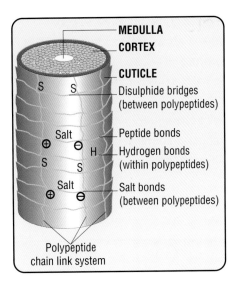

salt links

The **cortex** is the middle layer of the hair. It is by far the largest part of the hair and is the main source of the hair's strength. The cortex is where the changes take place during blow-drying, perming, relaxing, lightening and colouring.

The cortex is made up of many long strands of fibres, which resemble springs twisted together. The largest strands are the **cortical cells**, which are themselves made of smaller bundles called **macrofibrils**. These in turn are made up of bundles of **microfibrils**, and these in turn of bundles of **protofibrils**. All these fibres and cells are held together by **linkages** and **chains** which determine the hair's *elasticity*, *thickness*, *strength* and *curl pattern*.

The *colour* of the hair is determined by the **pigment**, which is also found in the cortex.

the medulla

The **medulla** is the very fine core of the hair. It does not have any real function and is not always present, particularly in fine blonde hair.

the chemical composition of hair

The cortical cells are made from **molecules** of **amino acids**. These are combinations of the elements **carbon**, **oxygen**, **nitrogen**, **hydrogen** and **sulphur**.

Amino acids are joined together by **peptide bonds**, forming long chains called **polypeptides**. These in turn form **proteins**.

The principal protein in hair is called **keratin**, and it is also found in the nails and the skin. Keratin has elastic properties which make the hair flexible and allow it to be stretched and curled without breaking.

Keratin chains are combined in hair in a coiled, spring-like shape. They are held in this shape by linkages *within* chains and *between* chains. There are three different kinds of linkage:
- disulphide bridges or sulphur bonds
- salt links
- hydrogen bonds.

The disulphide bridges are very strong linkages, but they can be broken and remade using chemicals during processes such as perming. It is this breaking and remaking of disulphide bridges that allows hair to be moulded to a new *permanent* shape.

The salt links and hydrogen bonds are much weaker, and are easily broken just with water. This allows the hair to be easily stretched and moulded, as when blow-waving. This change is only temporary, however, and the hair will return to its natural state when moisture enters. (See Chapter 6.)

the physical characteristics of hair

Hair is **hygroscopic**: it absorbs water from the atmosphere. The amount of water absorbed depends upon the **humidity** of the atmosphere – how dry or damp the *air* is – as well as how dry the *hair* is.

Hair naturally contains some moisture, which lubricates the fibres and allows the hair to stretch and recoil. Hair is also **porous**: it will absorb water like a sponge soaking up water. (This is called **capillary action**.)

Damaged hair is far more porous than healthy hair, and loses its natural moisture much more quickly. This is why it is more difficult to stretch and mould dry and damaged hair.

hair types

Caucasian or European hair

Mongoloid or Asian hair

Black or African-Caribbean hair

There are three different hair types, each of which can be of fine, medium or coarse textures:

■ **Caucasian** or **European** hair is mainly straight or lightly waved

■ **Black** or **African-Caribbean** hair has tight curls or kinks

■ **Mongoloid** or **Asian** hair is usually very straight and coarse.

cross-sections through hair: left, Mongoloid; centre, Caucasian; right, African-Caribbean

hair growth

Hair grows continually for a period of between about one year and six years. Each individual hair grows following a **cycle**, which includes a period of growth, rest and loss.

Eventually the hair falls out, but before it leaves the **hair follicle** (see page 15) a new hair is usually ready to replace it. If a new hair is not present an area of baldness will develop, as in male-pattern **baldness**. Normally, however, the cycle of growth is not really noticeable: because the hairs are all at different stages of growth, some are always in the growing stage.

stages of growth

There are three basic stages of growth.

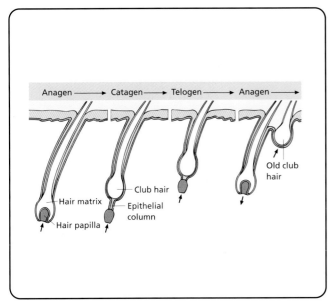

the hair growth cycle

- **anagen** This is the active growing stage of the hair growth cycle, which may last from about three months to several years.
- **catagen** This is the stage when the hair stops growing. It lasts for about two weeks. During this stage the hair separates from the **papilla** and begins to move up the follicle.
- **telogen** This is the resting stage. During this stage the follicle shrinks and separates from the papilla. This stage lasts for only a short period, after which a new anagen stage begins.

factors affecting hair growth

The healthy growth of new hair can be affected by many different factors. Here are some of the most common:

- poor health
- poor diet
- increasing age
- gender
- heredity
- hormones
- climate and environment
- physical treatment
- chemicals
- disease.

■ the skin

The skin is a complex organ which covers the whole of the body. Indeed, it is the largest organ of the body. It has many different layers and it performs several important functions.

protection

The skin provides a tough, flexible, waterproof covering which protects the underlying tissues from injury. It prevents harmful substances from entering the body unless the skin is cut, and contains a pigment called **melanin** which absorbs harmful ultraviolet rays from the sun.

The surface of the skin is itself protected by its natural oil, called **sebum**. This is mildly acidic (about pH 5.6) and has anti-bacterial properties which help prevent the growth of bacteria. Sebum also prevents the loss of water from the underlying layers of the skin, and so prevents the skin from drying out.

regulation of body temperature

The temperature of the body is regulated through **sweating**. Sweat evaporates and cools the surface of the skin.

excretion of waste

Waste products such as **water** and **salt** are removed from the body through sweating.

feeling

The skin contains **nerves** that allow the sensations of heat, cold, pain and touch to be experienced. These form a warning system that helps us to avoid harm and injury.

production of vitamin D

When exposed to sunlight, the skin produces **vitamin D**.

■ the structure of the skin

the epidermis

the epidermis

The **epidermis** is the layer of the skin nearest the surface. It is made up of five layers:

- ■ **the horny layer** This forms the outermost part of the skin. It has a hard surface, which is constantly being worn away and renewed by new cells. It takes about one month for cells to move up from the bottom of the epidermis to the top.

- ■ **the clear layer** This is a transparent layer, which contains the protein keratin.

- ■ **the granular layer** This contains granular cells. It is situated between the living cells below and the hardened dead cells above.

- ■ **the mixed layer** This contains a mixture of different live cells, including **prickle cells**, which lie just below the granular layer. The skin's colour pigment, **melanin**, is also to be found in this layer.

- ■ **the germinating layer** This lies at the bottom of the epidermis and is connected to the **basement membrane**, which is attached to the **dermis** (see below). It is the most active layer, where new epidermal cells are produced.

the dermis

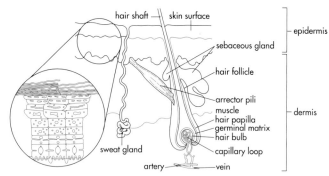

the hair in skin

The **dermis** lies in the middle part of the skin and is much thicker than the epidermis. It has a good supply of blood and is the source of nutrients for the skin.

- ■ **the reticular layer** The lower area of the dermis is composed of protein fibres which allow the skin to expand and contract.

- ■ **the papillary layer** The upper part of the dermis contains tiny projections called **papillae**, which contain the nerve endings.

the subcutaneous layer

The *subcutaneous layer* lies below the dermis. It is where the body stores *fat*.

the hair follicle

The *hair follicle* is the source of the hair's growth. Follicles are found all over the body, except on the lips, the palms of the hands and the soles of the feet.

At the bottom of the follicle is the *hair papilla* and a tiny group of cells called the *germinal matrix*. These are supplied with nerves and a good supply of blood to nourish cell growth. Hair is formed when the cells grow and move up the hair follicle. Gradually the cells harden and die, and the *hair* is formed. First the *hair bulb* is formed, then more cells are produced, and sooner or later they appear above the skin surface.

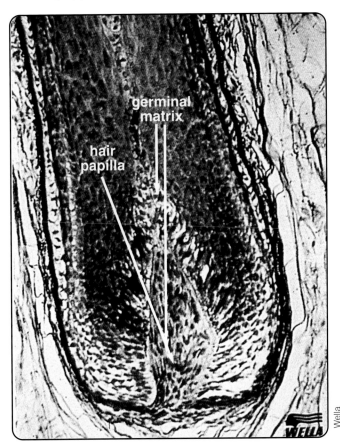

the hair papilla and the germinal matrix

the sweat gland

The *sweat glands* are found all over the body. They lie alongside each hair follicle and produce *sweat* which passes up onto the surface of the skin.

the sebaceous gland

Sebaceous glands or *oil glands* are found all over the body, except on the palms of the hands and the soles of the feet. They are usually situated alongside the hair follicle, which they open into: this allows their oil, *sebum*, to be secreted onto the hair and skin.

the arrector pili muscle

The *arrector pili muscle* is attached at one end to the hair follicle and at the other to the epidermis: when the muscle contracts, the hair stands erect. Together the erect hairs trap a layer of warm air around the body.

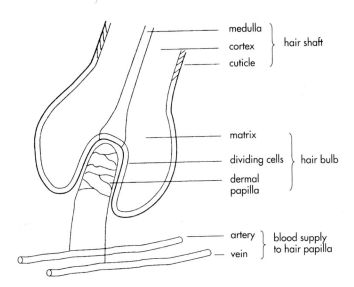

hair bulb

■ conditions of the hair and skin

bacterial diseases

condition	infectious?	cause	symptoms	treatment
furunculosis (boils and abscesses)	yes	Infection of the hair follicles by staphylococcal bacteria	Inflamed pus-filled spots with swelling and pain	By a doctor
sycosis barbae (barber's itch)	Yes	A bacterial infection of the hairy parts of the face	Small, yellow spots around the follicle, with irritation and inflammation	By a doctor
impetigo	Yes	A bacterial (staphylococcal or streptococcal) infection of the upper layers of the skin. Sometimes caused by shaving too close, which allows ingrown hairs to develop, which can become infected	Burning irritation with spots appearing, which become dry and crusted. The spots merge to form larger patches	By a doctor
folliculitis (inflammation of the hair follicles)	Yes	A bacterial infection, or sometimes chemical or physical damage	Inflamed follicles	By a doctor

Dr A. L. Wright

sycosis barbae

Dr M. H. Beck

impetigo

viral diseases

condition	infectious?	cause	symptoms	treatment
herpes simplex (cold sore)	Yes	A viral infection of the skin, possibly following exposure to extreme heat or cold, or reaction to food or drugs. The skin may carry the virus for many years	Irritation and swelling with inflammation, followed by the appearance of fluid-filled blisters, usually on and around the lips	By a doctor
warts and verrucae	Yes	A viral infection at the bottom of the epidermis, which causes the skin to harden and the skin cells to multiply	Raised, roughened skin, often brown or discoloured	By a doctor

fungal diseases

condition	infectious?	cause	symptoms	treatment
tinea capitis (ringworm of the head)	Yes	A fungal parasite, which infects the skin or hair	Circular areas of greyish white skin, each surrounded by a red ring. The hair is often broken close to the skin and it looks dull	By a doctor

infestations by parasites (infectious)

condition	infectious?	cause	symptoms	treatment
scabies	Yes	An allergic skin reaction to the presence of the itch mite, a small animal about the size of a pin head, which burrows into the skin, where it lays its eggs	A red rash, usually found in the folds of the skin between the fingers and on the wrists. It is very itchy	By a doctor
pediculosis capitis (head lice)	Yes	An infestation of the head by head lice	The lice can be seen by parting the hair, but more commonly the eggs (nits), or the empty egg cases, can be seen stuck to the hairs	By a doctor or with products available from chemists

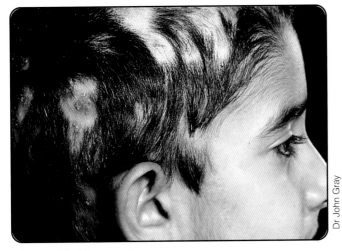

Dr John Gray

tinea capitis (ringworm)

Dr John Gray

pediculosis capitis

Dr. M. H. Beck

scabies

S. Lewis

head louse

disorders of the hair and skin

condition	infectious?	cause	symptoms	treatment
acne (a condition affecting the hair follicles and sebaceous glands)	No	Not known.	Spots or bumps, often seen on the face and forehead, which cause soreness, irritation and inflammation	By a doctor
alopecia (baldness or thin hair growth)	No	The hair follicles are not able to produce new hairs. The causes of alopecia are not fully understood but some forms, such as *alopecia areata*, may be brought on be stress. *Male-pattern alopecia* is hereditary. Pulling, such as when the hair is left in tight plaits for a long period, causes *alopecia traction. Cicatrical alopecia* is the result of scarring arising from physical or chemical damage to the follicles	Areas of baldness or thinning hair growth. Male-pattern alopecia often follows the Hamilton pattern	By a doctor or trichologist
canities	No	The colour pigment does not form in new hair growth – often associated with increasing age	White hairs are visible	Tinting
dandruff (pityriasis capitis)	No	A fungal infection, or through physical or chemical irritation	Small greyish-white flakes of skin	Many anti-dandruff medicines and shampoos are available
eczema and dermatitis	No	Physical irritation or an allergic reaction	The skin may be inflamed and split with weeping areas. There may be some irritation and pain	By a doctor
seborrhoea	No	Over-production of sebum, which may be due to physical or chemical irritants	Greasy, lank hair and greasy skin	Wash regularly using gentle massage movements and warm (not hot) water. A trichologist or doctor should treat extreme cases
psoriasis	No	Unknown	Patches of raised thickened skin, which may be red with silvery or yellow scales. The skin may be sore and/or itchy	By a doctor or a dermatologist

Dr John Gray

male-pattern alopecia – the hamilton pattern

Dr John Gray

alopecia areata

adverse conditions of the hair and skin

condition	infectious?	cause	symptoms	treatment
fragilitas crinium (split ends)	No	Physical or chemical damage	The ends of the hairs are dry and split	Remove the hair ends by cutting. Use a conditioner
monilethrix (beaded hair)	No	The hair develops irregularly while in the follicle	Bead-like swellings of the hair shafts, which often cause the hair to break close to the skin	By a doctor. Handle with care and use conditioner regularly
trichorrhexis nodosa	No	Physical or chemical damage	Patches of swelling and splitting on the hair shaft	Cutting and conditioning
sebaceous cyst	No	A blocked sebaceous gland	Bumps or lumps, about 10–50 mm across, on the scalp or nape	Removal of the cyst by a doctor
damaged cuticle	No	Physical or chemical damage	Rough areas of cuticle. The hair is dry and porous	Apply conditioners, thickeners or restructurants

Dr John Gray

psoriasis

Dr John Gray

trichorrhexis nodosa

Dr John Gray

damaged cuticle

Redken

fragilitas crinium (split ends)

health and safety

- If you suspect that an infectious condition is present, you must not proceed with the service. Seek advice from your manager or supervisor if necessary, and tactfully suggest that your client go to his doctor.

working safely

The barber must be able to recognise probable infections and infestations of the skin and hair in order to avoid catching them or passing them from one client to another. You must be especially alert to the dangers of two serious conditions that may be contracted through open cuts and abrasions.

AIDS

AIDS stands for *acquired immune-deficiency syndrome*. It is not a disease but a condition that makes the body more susceptible to diseases, and these may lead to death. To ensure that you protect your clients, your colleagues and yourself, you need to understand how AIDS is transmitted.

AIDS is caused by a virus known as the *human immunodeficiency virus* (*HIV*). People may carry the HIV virus – they are said to be 'HIV-positive' – without developing AIDS. However, a person who is HIV-positive could pass the virus to another person – but only if that person's infected body fluids, such as blood, come into contact with the other person's body fluids. Although this occurs most commonly through unprotected sex or when drug addicts share needles, the virus *can* be transferred through a cut or through broken skin.

The virus cannot live for long outside the body – you cannot catch it from toilet seats, for example.

hepatitis B

Hepatitis B is a disease affecting the liver. This too is caused by a virus, the *hepatitis B virus* (*HBV*). HBV is transmitted through infected body fluids such as blood, and also through infected water.

Hepatitis can affect the victim for a long time, and it can be fatal. Treatments are available, but the virus is known to be very resistant. It can survive a long time outside the body, so it is vital that you maintain a high standard of hygiene.

A vaccination is available to protect against hepatitis B. As a barber you are at risk from this virus, so you should consider having this vaccination.

■ health and safety

the need for hygiene

Effective hygiene is necessary in the salon to prevent infection and cross-infection, which may occur if the salon is dirty or if you or your client has an infectious condition or disease. *Cross-infection* usually occurs through physical contact with another person or via a tool, such as a razor, which has become infected.

The warm, humid atmosphere in the salon can be the perfect home for infectious organisms. *Sterilisation* with physical or chemical agents will destroy all the infectious and harmful micro-organisms, however, and *sanitation* will destroy some but not all micro-organisms. Regular cleaning with bleach or disinfectant will ensure that the risk of infection and cross-infection in the salon is minimised.

general salon hygiene rules

Always follow your salon's health and safety procedures.

- Cover any cuts or open wounds you may have, and ensure they remain covered.
- Maintain a high standard of personal hygiene. Wash your hands regularly.
- Use a clean gown and clean towels for each client.
- Be sure to clean and sterilise tools before using them on clients.
- Keep working surfaces clean. Sanitise them regularly using bleach or disinfectant.
- Store dirty laundry in a sealed container.
- Put waste in suitable bags that can be sealed. Contaminated materials and sharps must be stored and disposed of as specified by the local environmental health authority.

Martin Turner/S.F.T.W. Barbers Shop

interior of a barber's shop

Vidal Sassoon

3 cutting facial hair

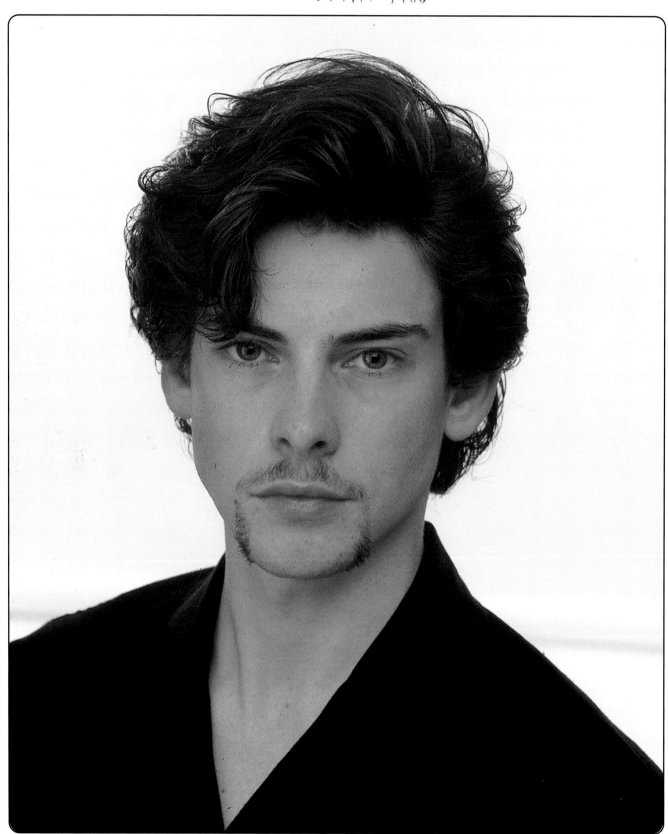

The **beard** and **moustache** have played an important role in men's fashions throughout the ages. At one time most men wore a beard, a moustache or long **sideburns**, but the popularity of the **clean-shaven** appearance increased following the introduction of safety razors and electric shavers. Today there is again a marked increase in the popularity of beards and moustaches, especially with young men, who now often wear short styles such as a goatee beard.

This chapter looks at the techniques used for cutting facial hair, and covers the following topics:

- cutting and styling facial hair – including traditional and current shapes
- consultation prior to cutting facial hair
- tools and equipment
- preparation for cutting facial hair
- cutting techniques
- a facial haircutting procedure
- finishing
- health and safety.

cutting and styling facial hair

The purpose of cutting facial hair is both to shorten the hair and to style it into shape. This is achieved with **scissors** or **clippers**, which are usually used with a **comb** to perform cutting techniques described as 'scissors-over-comb' or 'clippers-over-comb'.

Sometimes clippers are used with a **comb attachment** such that the hair is cut at a predetermined length. This attachment is relatively easy to use, and has become popular with many men for keeping their beards and moustaches in shape between salon visits.

traditional and current beard and moustache shapes

Over the years many beard, moustache and sideburn shapes have been developed. Some can be described as **traditional**, as men first started wearing them many hundreds of years ago. Some of these traditional shapes may also be described as being **current** shapes, because men today are still wearing the shape

or because the shape is currently fashionable. Yet other shapes are **new**, as they have only just been developed for the look that men like today: these too can be described as *current* shapes.

The barber must be familiar with many different traditional and current shapes, and able to visualise the right shape for each client and advise him accordingly. Here are some beard and moustache shapes for you to consider.

EXIT Hairdressing

Patrick Cameron

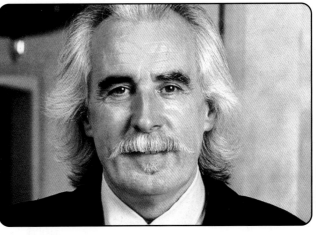

Charlie Miller

In the past beards, moustaches and sideburns would often be dressed into different styles using various *dressings*, *pomades* or *wax*. These made the hair very stiff and enabled the wearer to create intricate styles, such as the traditional *handlebar moustache*. *Dressing creams*, pomade, wax and *gels* are sometimes used to style facial hair today, but usually only to smooth stray hairs or to create definition or texture on longer beards.

a handlebar moustache

■ consultation prior to cutting facial hair

health and safety

■ Before you start cutting, you must carry out a thorough consultation. Be sure to identify any adverse conditions of the hair or skin that may be present. It is particularly important to establish whether you have reason to suspect any infection or infestation, as this would prevent you from cutting the facial hair. (This area is covered more fully in Chapter 2.)

When choosing the beard, moustache or sideburn shape it is important to consider the client's face shape and hairstyle. You should think of these as being integrated parts of one style, or one total look: choose a beard or moustache shape to suit.

Men are often very particular about their beard, so before you start work carefully consider each of the following factors.

■ What does the client want?

■ Why does he have, or wish to have, a beard or moustache?

■ Look for signs of broken skin, abnormalities on the skin, or any unusual facial features or beard growth patterns.

■ Is the beard hair fine, medium or coarse?

■ Is the beard growth dense or sparse? Does the density of beard growth vary around the face?

■ Pay attention to the client's face shape.

■ Pay attention to the length and shape of his hairstyle.

hair growth patterns

Hair growth patterns are the way in which individual hairs or a section of the beard may grow in a particular direction. Hair growth patterns must be identified because they determine both the shape that can be created and the techniques that you should use. Some clients have very strong hair growth patterns in their beard, such as *hair whorls*: these should be cut by following the direction of hair growth around the whorl.

tip

■ It is usually far better to go *with* the direction of beard growth than to go against it, especially when cutting strong growth patterns.

texture

The *texture* of hair in a beard can be fine, medium, or coarse. Young men usually have fine facial hair, but as men get older their facial hair often becomes much coarser. *Fine hair* is usually easier to cut, but some fuller styles will be more difficult to create. *Coarse hair* is often more difficult to cut, and is liable to fly in all directions during cutting – extra care must be taken to protect the client's and your own eyes. Coarser hair lends itself to many different beard shapes, but you must also consider the density of growth.

density

EXIT Hairdressing

Hair **density** is the amount of hair that grows in a given area of skin. Some men have a very dense beard growth, which is sometimes known as a **blue beard** because the density of growth gives the skin a blue tinge which remains even after shaving. Indeed, this could be the main reason why the client has grown a beard.

The density of beard growth often varies around the face. Some men have dense growth around their chin, cheeks and top lip, but sparse growth between the bottom lip and chin. Others have dense growth only on their top lip. Yet others have dense growth everywhere except on the top lip. And in others the density of growth may be very sparse, preventing the client from growing certain beard or moustache shapes.

tip

- Especially with new clients, it is particularly important when cutting existing beard shapes to look for variations in the density of growth: the hair may have been left long in some areas to disguise very sparse growth or to cover a scar. Cutting the hair too short in these areas would expose the skin, and might well annoy or embarrass the client.

health and safety

- Take extra care when cutting very coarse or dense beards. The hair is liable to fly in all directions while it is being cut. Make sure the client's eyes are well protected with clean cottonwool pads or tissues, and keep your own face well away from the work. If you find the hair is very strong and springy, you may need to wear safety glasses to protect your eyes.

face shape and facial features

It is important to identify the client's face shape and consider his facial features so that you can avoid damage to the skin and so that you can choose the most suitable shape. You must make careful note of the following:

- the size and position of the mouth
- the width of the top lip
- the shape of the nose
- the shape of the jaw and chin
- any unusual features, such as moles, dimples or scarring.

Different face shapes require different beard and moustache shapes. Here are some examples.

- **a round face** Choose a beard shape that is longer at the chin: this will make the face appear longer and less round. Keep the sides short and avoid bushy sideburns (which would make the face appear more round). A goatee beard is often a good shape to choose.

- **a large face** A larger moustache shape is usually more suitable: a small moustache would appear lost and would make the face appear bigger. The width of the top lip must also be considered: a large moustache would appear too big on a narrow lip.

- **a small face** The smaller face is more suited to smaller beard and moustache shapes.

- **a long face** Choose a beard shape that is fuller at the sides and shorter at the chin: this will help to make the face appear less long. Make sure any change in length is gradual, so as not to be obvious.

- **a square face** Full beard shapes are often more suitable. They should be shorter at the sides and longer towards the chin.

- **an oval face** Almost any beard shape is suitable, but you must take into account the client's hairstyle.

tips

- Use the mirror regularly during cutting to ensure that the developing shape is centralised and symmetrical.

- Pay particular attention to where the beard or sideburns meet the hairstyle, and ensure that they blend together.

tools and equipment

Read the section on haircutting tools in Chapter 4, 'Cutting men's hair' (page 44): this also applies to tools for cutting facial hair.

tools

All haircutting tools must be well-balanced, sharp, clean, and safe to use. Here are the main tools required for cutting facial hair.

scissors

Scissors are available in different sizes, ranging from 10 cm to 18 cm in length. Most barbers prefer scissors around 15 cm, but you need to find out what feels comfortable given the size of your hand and the job you are doing.

Thinning scissors are used to remove bulk without removing length.

clippers

Clippers may be either hand-operated or electric. **Hand clippers** are not usually used today unless electricity is unavailable, such as during a power cut.

Electric clippers may be powered by either mains electricity or rechargeable batteries. They are the preferred choice today because of their power, accuracy and convenience when compared to hand clippers. They are used to create outlines or when using clippers-over-comb techniques. Detachable **comb**

attachments are also available, which give a wide range of predetermined cutting lengths. These allow for very fast removal of hair and are sometimes used to reduce the length of the beard, which is then finished with scissors and clippers (without the comb attached).

razors

Razors are sometimes used to shave part of the face, to emphasise the beard or moustache style. **Disposable-blade razors** are best because they are more hygienic.

equipment

The client should be seated in an **adjustable chair** which can be positioned so that the client can recline comfortably. The chair should have a **headrest** and the height of the chair should be adjustable so that you do not have to bend uncomfortably.

preparation for cutting facial hair

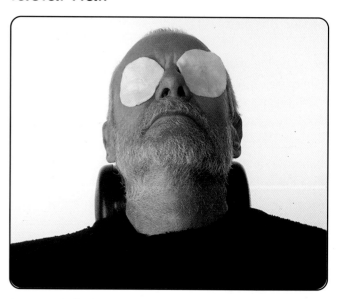

a prepared client

1 Carry out your consultation with the client. Look for signs of broken skin, abnormalities on the skin, and unusual beard growth patterns.

2 Determine the client's wishes and confirm what is to be done. Use photographs or pictures to help clarify the required shape.

3 Position the client in a reclining chair so that you can work on the beard. Ensure you provide support for his head.

4 Before you begin work, gather together all the tools and equipment you will need.

5 Gown the client and place a clean towel across his chest, tucked in at the neck.

6 Protect the client's eyes with tissue or cottonwool pads that have been moistened with warm water. The moisture helps the pads stay in place and will be soothing for the eyes. Make sure the tissue or pads are not *too* wet, however: they should be nearly dry.

7 Carefully comb the beard, disentangling the hair as necessary. Look out for areas of sparse growth, scarring or other unusual features you may not have seen earlier.

■ cutting techniques

The following cutting techniques are commonly used when cutting facial hair to shape.

scissors-over-comb

Scissors-over-comb cutting is performed by first lifting a section of hair, and then cutting straight across. When cutting beards and moustaches you should take small sections of hair: these are usually lifted with the comb as the hair is quite short. Some barbers, especially when working on longer hair, use the tips of their scissors to lift the sections of hair: the hair is then picked up on the comb and positioned ready for cutting.

Scissors-over-comb is often used to create graduated effects by adjusting the angle and length of each section. Be sure to use the fine teeth of the comb and the tips of the scissors when working around the lips.

clippers-over-comb

Clippers-over-comb cutting is often used instead of scissors-over-comb techniques, especially on longer, coarser and denser beards. Much the same effects possible with scissors can be achieved using clippers. Smaller clippers are easier to use on moustaches and when working around the lips, as the blades are smaller and more accurate.

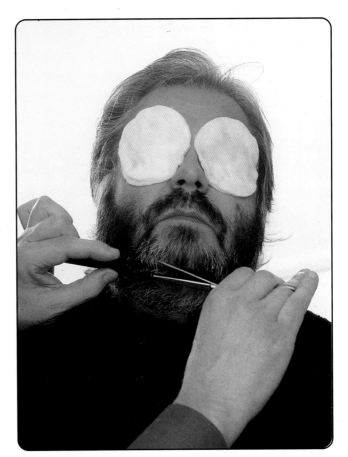

scissors-over-comb technique

freehand cutting

Freehand cutting is the cutting of hair without first taking the hair into a section or holding the hair in place with the comb or hand. It is often used to remove individual hairs or small amounts of hair when finishing a style, and is usually performed with the tips of the scissors. When cutting beards and moustaches it is used to smooth the outline shape and remove stray hairs.

razoring

Razoring is sometimes used to create clean outlines and emphasise a shape. It is performed with a razor, which may be either an open razor or a safety razor. *Disposable-blade razors* are best because they are more hygienic. *Electric razors* are also sometimes used.

■ a cutting procedure

the long beard

(a) before cutting | (b) starting at one side

1 Protect the client's clothes and eyes.

2 Comb the beard carefully, disentangling the hair where required.

3 Start at one side of your client (it does not matter which), and begin cutting the beard hair using the scissors- or clippers-over-comb technique (b). Start in the area where the sideburns join the head hair. Make sure you blend the beard and head hair to suit the overall look.

(c) cutting down the side | (d) cutting in the centre

4 Keep working down the side of the face (c), cutting the hair to the length determined by the chosen beard shape. Do not cut the moustache at this stage. If the beard is to be longer towards the chin you should gradually increase the length as you work down the beard.

5 Repeat this on the other side. As the shape develops, keep looking in the mirror to make sure that the beard is symmetrical.

6 Move to the centre of the beard and cut the hair using scissors- or clippers-over-comb techniques, as before (d). Take small sections, blending the two sides into the final shape. If you wish to create a pointed beard, angle your comb towards the point of the chin; otherwise blend the two sides together to create an even, continuous effect.

7 Move to one side of the moustache. Carefully outline the moustache along the top lip to create the required shape, using the tips of your scissors or the clippers (e). Use the fingers of your other hand to guide and support the scissors or clippers whilst cutting.

(e) outlining the moustache | (f) outlining the other side

8 Repeat this on the other side of the moustache (f).

9 Using your comb, lift small sections of the moustache hair and cut this to the required length. Use the tips of your scissors and small, careful movements (g).

10 Blend the moustache into the beard, as required by the overall shape.

11 Lift the client's chin and carefully cut the neck outline to the correct height (h). This outline may be graduated to create a natural effect, or cut into a clean line for a more defined look. The centre of the outline (below the chin) should be cut slightly higher than at the sides to compensate for the skin in the centre moving further up as the head goes back. The difference should be about 1 cm. This will appear level when the head is returned to its normal position.

12 Cut the other outlines on the cheeks, chin or above the moustache, as required. Refer to the mirror to keep the outlines symmetrical.

(g) cutting the moustache | (h) cutting the neck outline

13 Shave the areas outside the outlines if necessary (see Chapter 5).

14 Graduate the outlines to blend them with the skin, where required (i).

15 Finish the shape by combing the hair into place (j).

(i) graduating outlines

(j) the finished look

the short beard

(a) before cutting   (b) cutting the centre of the beard

1 Protect the client's clothes and eyes, as before (a).

2 Comb the beard carefully, disentangling the hair where required.

3 Start at one side of your client and begin cutting the beard hair, using the scissors- or clippers-over-comb technique or using a clipper attachment. Again, make sure you blend the beard and head hair to suit the overall look.

4 Keep working down the side of the face, cutting the hair to the length determined by the chosen beard shape. Do not cut the moustache at this stage. As with the long beard, if the beard shape is to be longer towards the chin you should gradually increase the length as you work down the beard.

(c) using clippers-over-comb for the centre of the beard   (d) cutting the moustache

(e) cutting the neck outline

5 Repeat this on the other side. Keep looking in the mirror to make sure that the beard is symmetrical.

6 Move to the centre of the beard and cut the hair, using scissors- or clippers-over-comb techniques or the clipper attachment (b). Blend the two sides into the final shape. If you wish to create a pointed beard, angle your comb towards the point of the chin; otherwise blend the two sides together to create an even, continuous effect (c).

7 Move to one side of the moustache. Carefully outline the moustache along the top lip to create the required shape, using the tips of your scissors or the clippers (d).

8 Repeat this on the other side of the moustache.

9 Using your comb, lift small sections of the moustache hair and cut this to the required length. The clipper attachment is not really suitable here.

10 Blend the moustache into the beard, as required by the overall shape.

11 Lift the client's chin and carefully cut the neck outline to the correct height (e).

12 Cut the other outlines on the cheeks, chin or above the moustache, as required. Refer to the mirror to keep the outlines symmetrical.

13 If necessary, shave the areas outside the outlines (see Chapter 5).

14 Graduate the outlines to blend them with the skin, where required.

15 Finish the shape by combing the hair into place (f).

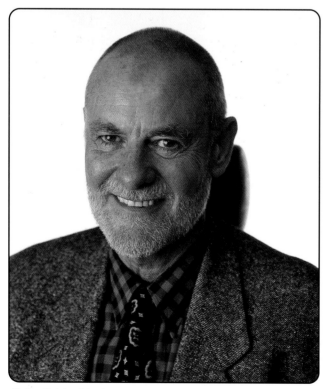

(f) the finished look

tip

■ The procedure for cutting a short beard into shape is basically the same as for cutting a long beard, but many barbers use a clipper attachment first to cut the beard to a predetermined length, and then finish with scissors and comb.

finishing

After cutting a styling aid may be applied to help smooth the hair, particularly on longer beard and moustache shapes. Use the mirror regularly to check the balance and symmetry of the shape as you dress it.

Comb the client's head hair into style, if required, and allow the client to see your work. Provide advice on after-care, as required.

health and safety

■ Always protect the client's eyes from hairs, which may fly up during cutting, especially on very coarse beards. Keep your own face away from your work; wear safety glasses for protection.

■ To ensure the client's comfort, remove excess hair cuttings from his face and neck at frequent intervals.

tips

■ When determining the correct height for the neck outline you should consider the overall shape and length of the beard. If the outline is too low it will be visible below the chin when viewed from the front: this can appear untidy. If it is too high, however, the outline will be visible across the side of the face. The best height is usually about 2 cm below the jawline, but always consider your client's wishes.

■ Outlines can be achieved by cutting the hair either with close-cutting clippers or with an electric razor. The outline hair may also be removed completely by shaving with a razor, which should be used following the shaving procedure described in Chapter 5.

■ health and safety

Everyone in the salon has a duty to work safely and keep the salon environment safe. When cutting facial hair it is important to consider health and safety because of the risks associated with using electricity and the risk of cutting the skin.

Here are some important health and safety factors that you must consider when providing haircutting services:

avoid infection

■ If the client has any cuts or abrasions on his face, or you suspect that an infection or infestation is present, you must not carry out the work.

■ Pay special attention to hygiene when cutting facial hair, because of the risk of cross-infection through open cuts.

■ Use only clean tools and equipment.

protect the eyes

■ Always protect the client's eyes from hairs using tissues or cottonwool pads. Keep your own face away from your work; if necessary, wear safety glasses.

work safely with razors

■ Open and safety razors have very sharp blades and must always be handled and used with great care.

■ When it is not being used or when it is being carried, always close the handle to protect the blade of an open razor.

■ Never place razors or other cutting tools in your pockets.

■ Always **sterilise** a fixed-blade razor before *each* use.

■ When using a detachable-blade open razor, always use a new blade for *each* new client.

■ Used razor blades, called **sharps**, must be disposed of correctly in accordance with your salon policy. Soiled disposable materials should be placed in sealed plastic bags for removal.

work safely with electricity

■ Always handle and use electrical equipment with care, and in accordance with the manufacturers' instructions.

■ Never place or use electric clippers or other electrical equipment near water.

■ Do not go near electrical equipment that is lying in water – first switch off the power at the mains.

■ Before commencing work, visually check that electrical equipment is safe to use. Check that the cable has not frayed or been pulled, and that the plug is not loose.

■ When using and storing electrical equipment, pay attention to the position of cables.

■ Never overload sockets. Do not plug too many items of electrical equipment into the same socket.

■ Follow the manufacturer's instructions for the care of your clippers. To avoid damage, be sure to clean and lubricate the blades regularly.

■ Electrical equipment must be regularly tested, and given a certificate of testing confirming that it is safe for use. The salon owner will ensure that this is carried out, as required.

be prepared for accidents

■ Make sure that you know the whereabouts of your salon's first-aid kit.

■ Keep yourself up to date with your salon's first-aid and accident procedures.

4 cutting men's hair

Competent *haircutting* is the foundation of all good hairdressing, and cutting skills are amongst the most important that any hairdresser has. These skills are particularly important to the barber because most clients visiting the barber's shop want their hair cut. Indeed, some barbers perform few, if any, other services.

This chapter looks at the techniques the barber uses for cutting men's hair. It covers the following topics:

- cutting and styling men's hair – including outlines, sideburns and neckline shapes
- consultation prior to cutting men's hair
- tools and equipment
- preparation for cutting men's hair
- cutting techniques – including wet and dry cutting
- cutting procedures
- finishing
- health and safety.

cutting and styling men's hair

The main purpose of cutting hair is to *style* the hair into shape. Both the hair length and the hair thickness can be removed, either to create a completely new look or just to trim the client's current look back into shape. Cutting also removes any *split ends (fragilitas crinium)* that may be present, thereby improving the condition and appearance of the hair.

Men's haircutting is achieved with *scissors* and *clippers*, although *razors* are also sometimes used as required to shave the outlines, thin the hair, or produce textured effects. *Club cutting* with scissors-over-comb and clippers-over-comb techniques is most often required.

Sometimes the clippers are used with a *comb attachment* that positions the blades to cut the hair at a predetermined length. These are particularly useful for creating short looks on longer hair, as the long hair can be removed quickly and easily to produce a rough shape ready for finishing.

Carl Shaw

Simon Shaw for WAHL

the haircut

The haircut has an important role in hairdressing because it is the basis on which all other hairstyling takes place. It determines how the hair can be later dressed and styled, and how easy that styling will be. A good haircut design should make the client look and feel good and will be easy for him to manage. Indeed, most men want a style that is 'easy to maintain'.

Lee Stafford

There are many similarities between cutting men's hair and women's hair. Often the same cutting techniques can be used and sometimes men and women wear the same looks, but there are usually subtle differences in the shapes that are required and in the methods that are used to achieve them. *Facial hair*, *dense hair growth* on the neck and *male-pattern alopecia* (baldness), which usually occur in men only, must be especially considered.

There are also distinct differences between masculine and feminine shapes. Masculine shapes are usually more square and angular and are suited to most men, while feminine shapes tend to be fuller and more rounded. Taller, less full, or leaner shapes are also more flattering on most men, so minimal thickness at the back and sides is often required. Remember that these are just basic principles, however: they should be adapted to take account of factors such as the client's wishes, his face shape and his hair growth patterns. The client consultation will help you determine which of these shapes is best suited to the particular client.

Most men, and many women too, wear short *layered looks*. These are popular because they require minimal blow-styling and dressing, and so are easy for clients to maintain. Many of these haircuts are so short that the styling details are quite subtle: precise cutting movements and accurate cutting angles are required. Often only very small amounts of hair are removed at a time until the desired effect is achieved – great care is

needed, as the hair is too short to hide any mistakes. Most short layered looks are *graduated* at the back and sides. The *outlines* of these haircuts are often emphasised, and these require careful attention.

cutting outlines

Many men have dense hair growth outside the natural hairline, particularly on the face and in the nape areas, whereas most women have soft, natural hairlines with few hairs growing outside. On women the outline usually requires little further definition, but on most men the haircut must be outlined or it appears untidy and unfinished.

In the past, *outlines* were cut with scissors and by shaving. The shaving was performed with an open razor and was used to remove all unwanted hair from outside the haircut outline. This produced a smooth, close finish that helped to extend the life of the haircut as the hair took longer to grow back. Today, outlines are usually shaped with the points of the scissors and with electric clippers, which can cut the hair nearly as close as when shaved. Shaving is still used sometimes, when a particularly close finish is required. Many barbers use both scissors and clippers throughout the outlining of a haircut. The choice of tool and technique is determined both by the needs of the haircut and by the barber's personal preference.

Simon Shaw

outlining with scissors

outlining with clippers

mutton chops

Here are some important points to remember about outlining men's haircuts:

- On most men the haircut must be outlined or it will appear untidy and unfinished.

- Follow the natural hairline wherever possible, particularly when outlining short haircuts. Avoid making unnecessary cuts into the natural hairline, especially around the ears and at the sides of the nape. (Such cuts would appear harsh and unnatural, and the haircut would soon appear untidy when the hair started to grow back.)

- Many outlines, particularly on shorter styles, appear more natural if they are gently tapered in the nape and at the bottom of the sideburns.

cutting sideburns

At one time most men wore a beard, a moustache, or long *sideburns*. The sideburns were often grown so long that they reached the bottom of the jawbone, and long distinctive sideburn shapes such as *mutton chops* became a prominent feature in men's fashion for many years. The introduction of the safety razor in about 1905 helped to establish the popularity of the clean-shaven appearance, and men started wearing their sideburns much shorter.

Today, sideburns are important in most men's haircuts, particularly on shorter styles because the sideburns are more visible. Many young men are now wearing longer sideburns, often shaped into points or other more elaborate designs. Most men, however, want sideburn shapes that are less prominent, with the emphasis on creating a natural, balanced look. The face

shape and the hairstyle should be used to determine the correct choice of sideburn shape for each client.

Here are some important points to remember about cutting sideburns:

- Most men's haircuts are improved by having sideburns. When cut to the correct length sideburns help to balance the haircut and create an attractive, masculine frame to the face.

- Avoid cutting the length of the sideburns higher than the top of the ear and into the hairline, as this creates a particularly harsh and unnatural effect. Men sometimes do this inadvertently when shaving, so offer advice on how to avoid this (see the tip below and Chapter 5, 'Shaving'). A drop of about 2 cm from the top of the ear is often acceptable, but remember to take into account other factors.

- Always ensure that the sideburns are cut level. Do not use the ears to determine the level of the sideburns, as they themselves are seldom level.

- Pay particular attention to where the haircut meets the sideburns and ensure that they blend together. You should think of these as being integrated parts of one style. Do not cut straight across the sideburns when outlining the haircut – this would produce a line across the sideburn through which the skin could be seen. The sideburns should be outlined by following down their natural hairline, adjacent to the ear.

levelling the sideburns

tip

■ To ensure that the sideburns are cut level, place the thumb of each hand high on each sideburn. Whilst looking in the mirror, slide one thumb down until the desired length is reached. Slide the other thumb down until both thumbs are level. Memorise the position of the thumbs – you can note a position on each ear as a point of reference. Now cut each sideburn to the correct length.

Consider sharing this tip with your clients, many of whom may have difficulty keeping their sideburns level when shaving.

Further information on cutting sideburns and other facial hair is provided in Chapter 3, 'Cutting facial hair'.

neckline shapes

a natural tapered neckline

The outline of the haircut in the nape is called the *neckline* shape. The neckline is important in men's hairdressing: the natural neck hairline is usually less well defined as hair often grows densely on the neck.

Over the years three basic neckline shapes have been developed to produce the looks that men like whilst ensuring that the haircut does not become untidy too quickly when the neck hair grows back. The three shapes are:

■ **squared neckline shapes** These are sometimes known as a *square cut*.

■ **tapered neckline shapes** These are sometimes known as a *taper cut*.

■ **rounded neckline shapes** These are sometimes known as a *Boston neckline*.

squared neckline shapes

cutting a squared neckline

Squared neckline shapes have clean distinct outlines that form a square shape. They can be achieved with scissors or electric clippers, which are often inverted and used to cut the neckline straight across. The neckline should be cut into a square corner where it meets the outline at the sides of the nape.

These outlines must be cut to follow the natural hairline, or a true square-cut shape will not be produced. Do not make any cuts into these outlines, as they would appear harsh and unnatural and the removed hair would soon grow back to make the haircut appear untidy. If required, the square-cut neckline may be gently tapered to produce a softer, more natural finish.

tapered neckline shapes

tapered neckline

Tapered neckline shapes have soft, graduated outlines that follow the natural hairline in the nape. They are far less severe than a squared neckline. The hair may be graduated through most of the back and sides of the head, or it may just be applied to the last few centimetres of hair at the bottom of the nape. Tapered necklines are usually achieved with scissors-over-comb and clippers-over-comb cutting techniques, though clipper attachments can also be used.

As with squared necklines, it is important that the outlines at the sides of the nape are cut to follow the natural hairline. Indeed, the whole neckline shape should still appear square, but without any distinct outlines.

rounded neckline shapes

rounded neckline

Rounded neckline shapes are similar to squared neckline shapes. They too have distinct outlines and appear square-shaped, but the corners of the neckline are then gently rounded. Rounded necklines can be achieved with scissors or electric clippers. Avoid making the shape too round, as rounded shapes are more feminine and are not usually suited to most men; also, any hair removed by such round shapes will soon grow back and make the haircut appear untidy. If required, rounded neckline shapes may be gently tapered to produce a softer, more natural finish.

tips

■ Cut the *sides* of the nape outlines before cutting *across* the neckline. This will help you to judge the proportions of the head and neck more clearly, and so determine the correct height at which to cut the neckline.

■ When cutting necklines, remember to take into account any hair growth patterns in the nape such as nape whorls, and ensure that these do not distort the required shape.

■ consultation prior to cutting men's hair

A successful haircut will always begin with a thorough consultation. The correct haircut design for each client relies on careful consideration of many different factors, which can only be identified through a consultation. Always make time to discuss the client's requirements and expectations with him, whether he is a new or a regular client.

Here are some of the critical factors you must consider when cutting men's hair.

■ Identify the client's requirements, then give him advice on suitable styles. Agree the final effect to be achieved.

■ Look for signs of broken skin or any abnormalities on the skin or hair.

■ Look for signs of any unusual hair growth patterns, and identify the natural fall of the hair.

■ Determine whether the hair is fine, medium or coarse.

■ Is the hair growth dense or sparse? Does the client have male-pattern baldness?

■ Is the client wearing an added hairpiece?

■ Does the client have a beard or a moustache?

■ Determine the features of the client's head, face and body. Is the client wearing spectacles or a hearing aid?

■ Take into account the approximate age of the client.

■ Consider the client's lifestyle.

health and safety

■ A thorough consultation will ensure that you identify any adverse conditions of the hair or skin that may be present. It is particularly important to establish whether a suspected infection or infestation is present: this would prevent you from carrying out the shave. (This area is covered more fully in Chapter 2, 'Client care for men'.)

hair growth patterns

Hair growth patterns are the way in which individual hairs or a section of the hair may grow in a particular direction. Hair growth patterns must be identified because they determine both the looks that can be created and the techniques that you should use. Some clients have very strong hair growth patterns: these need careful attention to produce the best effects, and sometimes just to prevent the hair from sticking straight up!

Here are some unusual hair growth patterns and the most suitable ways of cutting them.

double crown

With a **double crown** the hair is usually best left longer. If cut too short, the hair will stick up and will never lie flat.

nape whorl

A **nape whorl** may be found at either side of the nape, and sometimes at *both* sides. It can make the hair difficult to cut into a straight neckline – often the hair naturally forms a V-shape. Tapered neckline shapes may be more suitable, but sometimes the hair is best left long so that the weight of the hair overcomes the nape whorl movement.

cowlick

The **cowlick** is found on the hairline at the front of the head. It makes cutting a straight fringe difficult, particularly on fine hair, because the hair often forms a natural parting. It is usually better to cut the hair following this shape. Sometimes a fringe can be achieved by leaving the layers longer so that they weigh down the hair.

widow's peak

The **widow's peak** growth pattern appears at the front hairline. The hair grows upward and forward, forming a strong peak. It is usually better to cut the hair into styles that are dressed back from the face, as any fringe would be likely to separate and stick up. Short cropped styles or a parting may also be suitable, and sometimes a fringe is possible if the layers are left long.

a double crown

a cowlick

a nape whorl

Dr John Gray

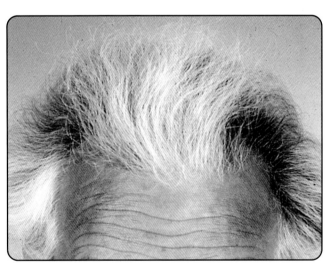
a widow's peak

texture

The **texture** of hair can be fine, medium, or coarse. **Fine hair** can be easy to cut, but some fuller styles will be more difficult to create and 'steps' are often more easily produced. **Coarse hair** can be more difficult to cut and is liable to fly in all directions during cutting, particularly on very short styles, so extra care must be taken to protect the client's and your own eyes. It is important when cutting very coarse hair to use sharp cutting tools and to take small cutting sections.

type

Hair **type** may be *tight curly*, *curly*, *wavy* or *straight*. Each hair type must be considered because the different types will behave differently when cut, so particular cutting techniques are more suited to some types than others. Here are some examples.

- **tight curly hair** Tight curly hair is often very difficult to cut with scissors-over-comb techniques, so scissors- or clippers-over-fingers and freehand

cutting techniques are mostly used. Razor-cutting is not usually suitable.

- **curly hair** Curly hair will coil back after being stretched during cutting, so remember not to cut it too short! Scissors- or clippers-over-comb techniques may be more difficult to use efficiently and accurately on curly hair, so cutting over the fingers is usually best.

- **wavy hair** Any of the cutting techniques can be used with wavy hair, but the position of the waves requires careful attention. Careful cutting is needed to ensure that the resulting wave movement suits the required look. Cutting the crests of the waves too short can make the hair stick up: dressing the hair into shape would then be difficult.

■ **straight hair** Straight hair – and especially fine straight hair – requires small, accurate sections to be used or marks and 'steps' may become visible. Straight hair may be cut with any of the cutting techniques, but razor-cutting on fine hair is usually not required.

density

Hair *density* is the amount of hair that grows in a given area of the scalp. It determines the choice of hairstyle that can be created and affects the techniques that are used.

baldness

Many people experience a noticeable reduction in the density of their hair as they get older. Common *baldness* is the most frequent cause of this hair loss. It can affect both men and women, but it is much more common in men. Indeed, about 50 per cent of men experience some hair loss by the age of 50, so many men must accept the likelihood of going bald, especially if their fathers have lost their hair.

Most baldness in men is caused by *male-pattern alopecia*. This is a hereditary condition in which some hair follicles stop producing terminal hairs and revert to producing vellus-type hairs. It is thought to result from the influence of the male hormone called *androgen*. The affected follicles usually follow a distinct pattern, the *Hamilton pattern* (page 18), which is seen in men throughout the world.

> **tip**
>
> ■ Before cutting the hair, especially with new clients, always look for signs of male-pattern alopecia or of alopecia areata: the hair may have been left long in some areas to cover the baldness. Cutting the hair too short in these areas would expose the skin, which would not go unnoticed!

The exact causes of male-pattern alopecia are still not fully understood, but over the years many different cures have been tried, usually with little success. Some men try to disguise the advanced stages of baldness by creating an unusually low parting in their remaining hair. The parted hair section is then grown long and combed up and over the bald area. This strategy is not particularly successful, as the section of hair may be many centimetres in length and is easily blown about when outdoors. Large amounts of sprays and dressings may be used to hold the hair in place, but the effect this creates is often unnatural and may simply cause the long strands of hair to be blown up together, exposing the scalp beneath and leading to considerable embarrassment.

> **tip**
>
> ■ The ends of the hair in the long hair section combed across the top of the head must be tapered and thinned to ensure that they blend in with the hair at the other side of the head. This is achieved with scissor tapering techniques applied to small sub-sections of the hair at a time. Use a slithering, backwards-and-forwards movement.
>
> Take great care not to cut the hair too short, or it will no longer reach the hair on the other side and the scalp will become visible. Never just cut this section of hair straight across: if you did, a harsh line would be clearly visible.

On most bald men, short layered looks and leaner haircut shapes are usually more flattering. These looks are more natural and more manageable, although men are often anxious about 'going short' on the first occasion, especially if they usually have long hair.

Dr John Gray

The impact of baldness on men should not be underestimated. During the consultation, handle this subject with great care. Always respect the client's wishes, especially with men who wish to retain the style with a low parting or who wear added hairpieces.

added hairpieces

Some bald men wear **added hairpieces** because they prefer the look that these create. Cutting a new hairpiece into shape is a specialist service that should be attempted only by those competent in this type of work. Further studies will be necessary if you are interested in acquiring these skills.

Some barbers specialise in providing such services and establish long and profitable relationships with their clients, but often the manufacturer or supplier of the hairpiece carries out this work. However, any barber will benefit by being able to *recognise* that an established hairpiece is worn and by knowing how to cut the client's natural hair to suit.

Here are some important things to remember about working with hairpieces.

■ **full hairpieces** Men who wear full hairpieces usually remove the hairpiece before visiting the barber's shop. They often have their natural hair cut short because it is not visible when the hairpiece is worn.

■ **smaller hairpieces and toupees** Some barbers leave smaller hairpieces and toupees in place while they cut the client's natural hair. The hairpiece hair is sectioned at the bottom and held out of the way with cutting clips to gain access to the natural hair beneath. (Do not use brightly coloured butterfly clips – these would certainly embarrass the client.) This method of cutting is sometimes preferable because it allows the barber to determine the correct length at which the natural hair should be cut and so blend the hairpiece in more effectively. Scissors-over-comb cutting techniques are used, and great care must be taken as any cuts to the hairpiece will not grow back!

■ **removing hairpieces** Hairpieces are usually held in place by special double-sided sticky tape. They should be removed by the client himself, to avoid causing any discomfort.

tip

■ If the client wears **spectacles** or an external **hearing aid**, ask him to remove them while you cut his hair, but remember to take them into account during cutting. Some spectacles may cause the hair to stick out if it is not cut correctly. Hearing aids often clip over the back of the ear, and the client may wish you to leave the hair longer to disguise them.

tip

■ If the client has a beard or moustache you must think of these as being integrated parts of one style. Choose a haircut shape to suit the total look.

features

The features of the client's head, face and body must all be noted to ensure that you choose the most suitable haircut shape. Every haircut should be designed to suit the head and face shape. Your decisions about the hair length, thickness and balance must all relate to the features of these underlying structures.

Careful consideration must be given to each of the following:

■ the shape of the face – round, square, oblong, long, short, or whatever

■ the size and position of the ears

■ the size and shape of the nose

- the shape of the jaw and chin
- any unusual features, such as a high front hairline
- the way the head and body are held
- the length and width of the neck.

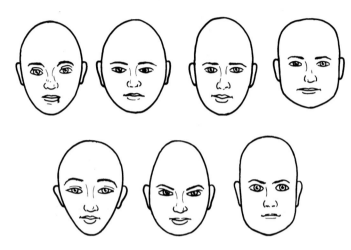

face and head shapes

Different head and face shapes require different haircut shapes. Here are some examples.

- **a round face** Choose a haircut shape that is dressed higher at the front and top. The sides should be less full, or leaner. Avoid full, round shapes, as they would make the face appear more round.

- **a large head and face** A large, full haircut shape may be more suitable, as a small shape can appear lost and out of proportion, but the shape of the face must also be considered.

- **a small head and face** The smaller face is more suited to less full, leaner haircut shapes: the face would appear swamped by large, full and fussy styles.

- **a large nose** Fuller shapes with side partings usually help to diminish a large nose. Avoid centre partings and dressing the hair straight back off the forehead.

- **a tall person** Taller shapes accentuate the person's height, so flatter shapes are better.

- **a short person** Flatter shapes will make short people appear shorter, so taller shapes are usually best.

- **a long face** Choose a shape that is fuller at the sides and shorter on the top. This will help to make the face appear less long.

- **a square face** Taller shapes are often more suitable. They should be short and less full at the sides, but longer and higher towards the top.

- **an oval face** An oval face shape is considered to be the ideal because most haircut shapes will suit it. Remember to take into account the client's other features, however, such as the position of his eyes and ears.

tip

- Use the mirror regularly during cutting to ensure that the developing shape is balanced.

age

The client's age must be considered because people of different ages usually require different hairstyles.

- **children** Children mostly require simple hairstyles that need little or no dressing and styling, so shorter styles are often best.

Regis

■ **teenagers** Teenagers wear many different styles. Some of these are common to older age groups, but many young men want highly personalised styles. This age group is often prepared to carry out daily grooming, blow-styling and dressing to achieve their chosen look. Distinctive and sometimes quite extreme looks are required, which may be either short or long.

■ **young men** Young men usually require fashionable but practical styles which are easy to manage and are in keeping with their chosen style of clothing. Preferred styles are often similar to those worn by teenagers, but usually less extreme.

JFK Edinburgh for Goldwell

Daniel Hill

Charles Worthington

Vidal Sassoon

■ **mature men** Mature men usually require practical styles that are easy to maintain. Shorter shapes are most popular.

lifestyle

The client's *lifestyle* also affects the choice of haircut design. Busy men may not have the time to look after fussy styles; long hair may not be suitable for those who take part in a lot of sport, as drying the hair can take too long. Particular jobs sometimes require particular haircuts – for example, short haircuts are required for those in the army, fire service or police.

Vidal Sassoon

■ tools and equipment

tools

All haircutting tools must be well-balanced, sharp, clean and safe to use. Here are the main tools required for cutting men's hair.

scissors

Scissors are available in different sizes, ranging from 10 cm to 18 cm. Barbers usually prefer scissors around 15 cm in length, but it depends on what feels comfortable in the size of your hand and for the job you are doing.

Haircutting scissors should be held with the thumb through one handle and the third finger through the other. Only the blade that is operated by the thumb should move when the scissors are being used. This method will produce the most accurate results and it provides the most control and stability, which is vital when cutting around delicate areas such as the ears.

Good-quality hairdressing scissors can be quite expensive, but they will last you for many years if you look after them. Only ever use them for cutting hair, or they will quickly become blunt. Keep them clean, and always remove loose hairs, grease and any dirt before disinfecting or sterilising them. Never use dirty scissors because of the risk of passing infection from one client to another.

Clean and lubricate the scissors regularly, and especially before using them on each new client. Many different disinfectants, alcoholic wipes and disinfectant sprays are available for this purpose.

Thinning scissors are used to remove bulk without removing length. The blades are serrated so that when the blades are closed only some of the hairs are cut. One or both of the blades may be serrated, and scissors are available with different numbers and sizes of serrations. The size and number of the serrations determine how many hairs are cut when the blades are closed.

thinning scissors

clippers

Clippers may be either hand-operated or electric. *Hand clippers* are operated by squeezing the handles together. They are seldom used today unless there is no access to electricity, such as during a power cut. *Electric clippers* may be powered by either mains electricity or rechargeable batteries, and are operated by an electric motor or a magnetic coil.

detachable-blade electric clippers

Electric clippers are the preferred choice today because of their power, accuracy and convenience in comparison with hand clippers. They are available in three different designs and with a range of different blade sizes for different purposes. The *number 000* blade is good for removing hair from outside the outlines, whilst the *number 1* blade is best for clipper-cutting the hair to remove bulk.

Here are the most common sizes available.

	blade sizes	cutting length of blade
detachable blades The blades are available in a wide range of sizes.	0000	A very close cut (similar to shaving)
	000	0.3mm (a close cut)
	00	0.4mm
	0	0.8mm
	0A	1.2mm
	1	3.3mm
	1A	4.0mm
	11/2	4.8mm
	2	6.4mm
	3	7.9mm
adjustable blade Moving a small lever alters the cutting length of the blade. (Hand-operated clippers often have adjustable blades.)	From 000 to 1	As above
non-adjustable blade	A fixed setting between 000 and 1	As above

adjustable-blade electric clippers

tip

■ Develop your skills by using the scissors before you start cutting any hair. A good exercise is to open and close the scissors several times whilst moving up along a flat vertical surface. Concentrate on making the thumb blade move whilst keeping the other blade still. Make the movements slowly at first – increase the speed only when you become more proficient.

Detachable comb attachments are also available for electric clippers, which give a wide range of predetermined cutting lengths. These allow for very fast removal of hair and are sometimes used to reduce the length of the hair and produce a rough shape, which is then finished with scissors and clippers (without the comb attached). The combs are available in sizes ranging from a **number 8**, which will leave the hair about 25 mm long, to a **number 1**, which will leave the hair only about 1 mm long after cutting. The most popular sizes are the **number 3**, which leaves the hair about 10 mm long, and the **number 4**, which leaves the hair about 13 mm long.

health and safety

■ Before using the clippers, and especially after cleaning the blades, always check that the top, movable cutting blade is not protruding beyond the lower, static blade. If the movable blade protrudes it would cut the client's skin.

razors

Razors are used in men's haircutting to shave outlines, to thin and style the hair, or to produce textured effects. **Disposable-blade razors** are preferable because they are more hygienic, but **open razors** are also sometimes used. Detailed information on razors is provided in Chapter 5, 'Shaving'.

combs

Combs are available in various different sizes for different purposes. Cutting combs are usually thin and pliable, with fine teeth at one side and coarse teeth at the other. The **coarse teeth** should be used for most combing and sectioning, while the **fine teeth** are good for detailed work and close cutting. The **barber comb** is specifically designed for this purpose. It is very thin and pliable and the side with the fine teeth narrows to a point. This makes the comb easier to use when producing fine tapered finishes, especially in confined areas, such as around the ears.

A cutting comb should fit comfortably in the hand and be easy to move into all the positions required during cutting.

neck brush

A **neck brush** is required to remove excess hair cuttings and to maintain the client's comfort throughout the service.

equipment

The client should be seated in an **adjustable chair** (see pages 78-9), which can be positioned at the correct height so that the hair can be worked on efficiently.

■ preparation for cutting hair

1 Carry out your consultation with the client.

2 Determine the client's wishes and confirm what is to be done. Use photographs or pictures to help clarify the required shape.

3 Before you begin work, gather together all the tools and equipment you will require.

4 Gown the client, placing a clean tissue or neckstrip between the client's neck and the gown. A cutting collar may then be placed on top of the gown. Some barbers use a clean towel instead of a cutting collar, particularly if the hair is wet. This should be placed across the client's back and be tucked in at the neck.

5 Position the client in a chair so that the hair can be worked on efficiently.

6 Carefully comb the hair, disentangling it if required. Look out for areas of sparse growth, scarring or other unusual features you may not have seen earlier.

■ cutting techniques

Vidal Sassoon

The techniques used for cutting men's hair are generally the same as those used in women's hairdressing. The barber understands, however, that differences exist in the way the techniques are used and in the effects they achieve.

The following cutting techniques are commonly used when cutting men's hair.

club cutting

In **club cutting** the sections of the hair are cut straight across to produce blunt ends which are all cut at the same length. Small sections are required, particularly on coarse, dense hair, or the hair ends will not be level. This technique may be used on wet or dry hair.

Here are the main methods of club cutting used in men's hairdressing.

scissors-over-comb

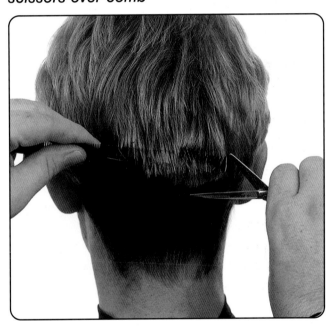

scissors-over-comb technique

The **scissors-over-comb** technique is performed by lifting a section of hair and then cutting it straight across. When cutting short hairs in the nape you should take extra-small sections of hair, which are usually lifted with the comb. Some barbers use the tips of their scissors to lift the longer sections of hair, which are then picked up on the comb and positioned ready for cutting. Ensure that you use the coarse teeth of the comb and the main part of the scissors when cutting the interior of the haircut, and the fine teeth and the tips of the scissors when working around the ears and nape.

Scissors-over-comb is mostly used on shorter styles, particularly to create graduation in the nape and at the sides.

clubbing over the fingers

clippers-over-comb technique

clubbing over the fingers

Clubbing over the fingers is very similar to the scissors-over-comb technique – indeed, it might be called 'scissors-over-fingers'. It is performed by lifting a section of the hair, which is then combed out and transferred to the fingers. The fingers slide up the section of hair to the correct position for cutting, and the hair is then cut straight across. The hair may be held at different angles, and different sizes of sections may be used, to create the amount of graduation required.

Clubbing over the fingers is mostly used on longer styles and to cut the top of many short styles.

clippers-over-comb

Clippers-over-comb can be used instead of scissors-over-comb and clubbing-over-the-fingers techniques, especially on long, coarse and dense hair, and particularly if it is being taken much shorter. Much the same effects possible with scissors can also be achieved using clippers. Clippers are best used on dry hair.

freehand cutting

Freehand cutting is the cutting of hair without first taking the hair into a section or holding the hair in place with the comb or hand. It is often used to remove individual hairs or small amounts of hair when finishing a style, or for producing textured effects. It is usually performed with the tips of the scissors.

Freehand cutting can be particularly useful when cutting tight curly or curly hair, and is often used on beards and moustaches to smooth the outline shape and remove stray hairs. Tapered effects can also be achieved freehand by using sliding and slicing movements.

tight curly hair

tapering

Tapering is used to cut the hair so that it tapers to a point. Both unwanted weight and unwanted length may be removed. Tapering is particularly useful for blending in heavier sections of the hair, as the weight at the ends can be reduced without affecting the hair length.

Here are some methods that are commonly used in tapering men's hair.

scissor tapering

razor tapering

scissor tapering

Scissor tapering (sometimes called *slithering*) is carried out on dry hair. It is achieved by moving the open scissor blades backwards and forwards along the hair section in a slithering, sliding movement. The blades are gently opened and closed a small amount during the movement, to remove just the required amount of hair. The blades must not be *completely* closed or the section of hair will be cut straight through.

razor tapering

Razor tapering is used only on wet hair. It is achieved by placing the razor on the hair at an angle of about 30–40°, and then making gentle slicing movements with the razor such that it cuts the hair.

On shorter hair, the section to be cut should be combed through until the comb is at least 3 cm away from the hairline. The comb is then kept in this position and the razor is placed at the correct angle on the hair, about 2–3 cm down from the comb. The hair is cut using gentle slicing movements with the razor. The razor and comb should move down the section together, remaining about 2–3 cm apart throughout.

tip

- Take great care when cutting with a razor. Do not razor-cut the hair too near to the hairline or roots: if you do, it will stick up and be very difficult to style. Always use *gentle* cutting actions and small movements – if used incorrectly, the razor will quickly and easily remove too much hair!

Simon Shaw

Charles Worthington

health and safety

- Razors have very sharp blades and must always be treated with care and respect. Keep the handle closed or cover the blade when not in use, and especially when carrying or passing a razor. Never place a razor in your pockets, and always keep razors out of the reach of children.

thinning

Thinning techniques are used to remove bulk and thickness without affecting the overall length. Thinning is achieved by cutting just *some* of the hairs in a section of hair, while leaving others uncut so that the length of the overall section remains unchanged. The hair should be cut only in the middle third of the section: if it is cut too close to the roots, the resulting short hairs will stick straight out.

Here are the most common methods used for thinning men's hair.

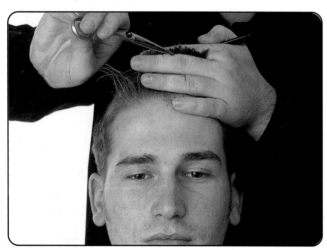

scissor thinning

scissor thinning

Scissor thinning is achieved using a similar action to that used in scissor tapering, but here the open scissor blades are moved along the hair section in one long movement. The hair may also be cut with the points of the scissors, known as *point cutting* or *pointing* – this technique should be used in the middle of the hair section. Sometimes it is used to thin the ends of the hair and to create softer lines.

cutting with thinning scissors   thinning with a razor

cutting with thinning scissors

Thinning scissors have serrated blades: when closed, they cut only some of the hairs. They should be used in the middle third of the section or towards the ends.

thinning with a razor

Thinning with a razor is carried out only on wet hair. It is achieved by placing the razor on the hair at an angle of about 30–40° and then cutting the hair by gentle slicing movements. Gentle actions are required or the hair will be cut straight through!

texturising

Texturising techniques are used to break up a solid mass of hair to give a more random movement and texture. Many different cutting techniques can be used to produce the varying lengths of hair that create the 'textured' effect. Usually freehand *pointing*, *chipping*, *slicing* and *chopping* actions with the scissors will produce the required effects. The razor can also be used to achieve similar effects.

texturising: chipping with scissors

Simon Shaw

texturising: pointing with scissors

Many men have **natural partings**. To identify these, comb the wet hair straight back, then push it forward with the palm of the hand: where the hair parts naturally is the natural parting. Such partings should be used, where possible, as the resulting style will be easier to manage. The natural hair growth patterns and the hair fall must all be identified and considered to determine where, if at all, a parting is required.

The hair is usually cut in the middle third of the section and towards the ends, as cutting too near the roots will make the short hairs stick out. Short layered haircuts are often texturised through the top to disconnect the shape and create a sensation of movement and energy.

partings and fringes

partings

fringes

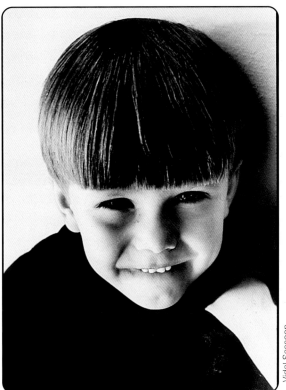

Vidal Sassoon

The front of the hair may be dressed into a **fringe**. Men do not often wear full fringes, but many children do. A fringe shape may be short, long, squared, rounded, blunt-cut or tapered.

The client's head and face shape will determine which fringe shape is best. The fringe should not be too heavy or it will appear unnatural, and fringes can even look like artificial hair! Layering is often used to reduce the thickness, and the ends are sometimes tapered to produce a softer line. Hair growth patterns such as a cowlick or widow's peak must be considered as they may make a full fringe impractical. Remember that it is usually better to go *with* the natural hair fall rather than *against* it.

Many men's hairstyles have **partings**. These can be used in many different ways and to create many different effects. For example, partings may be used to draw attention away from unwanted prominent facial features, such as a large nose or large ears. Centre partings and side partings are often used to divide large hair masses and produce more pleasing and symmetrical shapes, which are also more manageable.

wet and dry cutting

Traditionally, most men visited the barbers' shop to have their hair cut dry. A dry cut produced good results and was completed more quickly than a wet cut. Today, many men have their hair washed and then cut wet, but dry cutting is still common.

If the client's hair is greasy and dirty then it must be washed before you can cut it. Wet hair is also required for blow-styling and some cutting techniques, such as razor-cutting, which should always be carried out on wet hair to avoid causing damage to the hair and discomfort to the client. Other cutting techniques are less suitable for use on wet hair, such as some scissor-tapering and clippers-over-comb movements. In general, *scissors* can be used on wet or dry hair, *razors* must only be used on wet hair, and *thinning scissors* and *clippers* are best used on dry hair.

> ### tip
> ■ If you wish to carry out dry cutting, it is best to wash and dry the hair first. Be sure to explain this to the client first and take his wishes into account.

> ### tip
> ■ Remember that hair stretches by up to half its own length when wet. Keep this in mind when you are cutting stretched hair, so that it is not too short when it dries.

layering

The purpose of **layering** is to produce a series of connected, unbroken layers, with no perceptible lines or 'steps' in between. Most men wear layered haircuts: these often produce a more masculine shape and are easier to manage.

Here are the two main layered effects that are mostly required in men's hairdressing.

uniform layering

uniform layering

Uniform layering is the process of cutting the sections of the hair to the same length. It can be achieved by holding each section at 90° to the head, and then cutting the hair straight across at the same angle.

Uniform layering is used mostly in longer styles, and to cut the hair on the top of the head in some shorter styles. It is particularly suitable for creating shapes on curly hair.

graduated layering

graduated layering

Graduated layering is the process of producing a difference in length between the layers at the top and the layers at the bottom of a section of hair. This can be achieved by elevating the sections of the hair at different angles and then cutting them straight through, or by holding the sections at 90° to the head and then cutting through the section at a different angle. Lifting the sections *higher* and then cutting them will produce a *greater* amount of graduation; holding them *lower* and then cutting will produce *less*.

The gradient between the top and bottom of the hair sections when positioned back on the head is called the *angle of graduation*.

- If you hold a section of hair at 90° (a right angle) to the back of the head, and cut it at 90° to the section, you will produce a 45° angle of graduation.
- If you hold a section of hair at 90° and cut it at 45° you will produce a steeper graduation.
- If you hold a section of hair at 90° and cut it at 145° you will produce a *level length*, in which all of the ends of the hair fall level, without graduation.

producing a level length

producing a 45° angle of graduation

producing a 20° angle of graduation

Many men's haircuts are graduated at the back and sides to produce taller, leaner, more masculine shapes.

cutting guidelines

The *cutting guideline* is the line that is created by the ends of the hair when a section of hair is held out from the head. Establishing correct guidelines is very important when cutting the hair: if this is not done, the results will be uneven and inaccurate, and will not be likely to meet the client's requirements.

Some cutting guidelines are called the *baseline* or *perimeter line*. These are used to determine the outer and inner perimeters of the haircut. These lines are important because they usually provide the basis for the other guidelines to follow.

To produce precise, accurate results, the guidelines should be carefully followed throughout the cutting process. Make sure that a guideline from a previously cut section of hair is clearly visible before cutting the new section of hair. Both the hair length and the line of the cut in the previous section should be used to guide where the next cut is to be made.

When preparing guidelines, many different factors must be considered – the position of the ears, the nose and the eyes, the shape of the head and the position of the hairlines, and so on. During the cutting process the head is often divided into large sections, rows or panels, to ensure that the guidelines are easily seen and to make the hair more manageable. Each of these sections or panels is then sub-divided into sections of hair for cutting. The cutting guideline established in one section is transferred from section to section, and panel to panel, so that the resulting haircut is connected throughout to produce an even result.

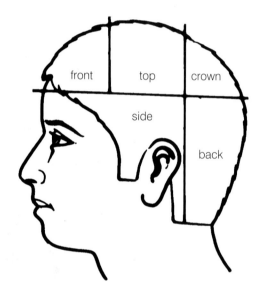

guide sections

In men's hairdressing, particularly on shorter styles, the head is often divided into three main areas, which reflect the different shapes that are required and the techniques that are used.

■ Area 1 includes the hairline, the ear outline and the occipital bone. This is where most of the graduation and tapering is carried out. Usually scissors- or clippers-over-comb techniques are required.

■ Area 2 is between the occipital bone and the bottom of the crown area. On shorter styles this is where the graduation and taper are blended into the hair in the top section. Thickness is often reduced here to create the taller, less full, more masculine shapes that most men prefer. Usually scissors- or clippers-over-comb and over-fingers techniques are required.

■ Area 3 covers the rest of the top of the head, starting from the crown area. The blending of area 2 continues, and the lengths of the top and front are determined. Scissors- or clippers-over-comb cutting techniques can be used, but more often scissors- or clippers-over-fingers techniques are required.

guide sections

■ cutting procedures

In cutting men's hair, several different *cutting procedures* may be followed. Each individual barber will decide where to start and which cutting techniques to use, mainly according to personal preference.

Many different cutting techniques can achieve similar effects. They can also be combined and adapted as necessary, to achieve the required results. The best procedure is one that allows the barber to work accurately and efficiently throughout the whole haircut.

The following examples show how some common men's looks can be achieved.

short layered looks

a tapered neckline

(a) before cutting   (b) starting at the back

Simon Shaw

1 Protect the client's clothes.

2 Comb the hair carefully, disentangling it where required (a).

3 Start in the centre panel of hair at the back of the head and begin cutting the hair (b). If using the clippers, choose the comb attachment for the length of cut you require. (The best size of comb for this look is either a number 3 or a number 4.) Ensure that the comb is securely attached to the clippers. A scissors- or clippers-over-comb technique may be used instead, if preferred.

4 Place the clippers flat against the neck, just below the neckline. Using a *smooth continuous movement*, push the clippers slowly up the head, keeping them flat against the scalp until you reach the area where you want the taper to begin. In a smooth *rocking* movement, *pivot* the clippers away from the head to produce the shape and length of hair that you want. Unless the top panels are to be cut short as well, *do not go higher than the occipital bone* without pivoting away from the head.

5 Move to the adjacent panel of hair and repeat the process as before. Make sure you follow the cutting guideline from the previous section and the adjacent panel. If the panels are not connected, long hairs will be left between them.

6 Keep working around the head, cutting the hair to the length determined by the chosen haircut shape. Do not cut the sides at this stage, if the hair is to be longer around the ears. Gradually increase the length of the hair by pivoting the clippers away as you work towards the sides (c).

7 Repeat this on the other side. As the shape develops, keep looking in the mirror to make sure that it is symmetrical. Consult with your client at regular intervals to confirm that the developing shape is correct, making adjustments if required.

(c) cutting the sides   (d) shaping the sideburns

8 Remove the comb attachment from the clippers. Move back to the centre panel of hair at the back of the head. Using either scissors- or clippers-over-comb techniques, begin to blend the hair where the top of the taper meets the hair on the top of the head. Move across the head, taking small sections. Ensure that the panels are connected, blending areas together to create an even, continuous effect.

9 Move to one side of the head. If your client has sideburns, note the required length. Carefully outline the sideburn and the hair around the ears (d, e), then move down the sides of the nape with the tips of your scissors or with the clippers. Use the fingers of your other hand to guide and support the scissors or clippers whilst cutting.

(e) outlining hair round the ears   (f) levelling the sideburns

10 Repeat this on the other side of the head. Ensure that the sideburns are level (f: see the tip on page 36). As you create the outlines, *make sure you do not cut into the natural hairline, particularly at the sides of the nape* (g).

11 Position the client's head so that it is bent forward slightly. Carefully cut the neckline to the correct height. Use the proportions of the head and neck, the length of the hair and the position of the ears to determine the length that is most suitable. The neckline must be tapered to create a natural effect: do not cut it straight across. Use scissors-over-comb or clippers-over-comb techniques. The bottom edge of the comb should be held against the skin, then angled so that the hair will be cut shorter at the bottom and left longer at the top (h).

(g) outlining the nape   (h) tapering around the neckline

12 Move to the top of the head and take a section of hair at the crown (i). Using the clubbing-over-fingers technique, with either the scissors or clippers, cut the hair to the required length. Move across the head, taking small sections, and ensuring that successive panels of hair are connected, as before (j, k).

13 Blend the top panels and the side and back panels where they meet, to create an even, continuous effect (l).

14 Texturising techniques may be used through the top, as required (m, n).

(i) taking a section at the crown   (j) clubbing the top

(k) clubbing the top   (l) blending the top with the sides and back

Simon Shaw

15 Shave the areas outside the haircut outlines, if necessary (see Chapter 5).

16 Graduate the outlines to blend them with the skin, where required.

(m) texturising   (n) texturising

17 Finish the shape by combing, styling and dressing the hair into place (o).

(o) a finished look

Simon Shaw

alternative finished looks

Simon Shaw

tip

■ Before cutting the hair, make sure that you can clearly see the cutting guideline created by the previous section. If the hair is too thick for you to see the guideline through it, you may need to take a thinner section.

a squared or rounded neckline

The procedure described is for a **squared neckline**. For a **rounded neckline**, follow this sequence and after the squared shape has been created, simply round off the corners of the neckline.

1 Protect the client's clothes.

2 Comb the hair carefully, disentangling it where required (a).

(a) before cutting   (b) cutting a section at the crown

3 With the hair wet, section the hair in two by making a parting from ear to ear across the top of the head. Take a section *parallel* to this parting at the crown and hold it at 90° to the head (b). Cut this section straight across to the correct length using the scissors-over-fingers technique.

4 Take a section going down the centre panel towards the front hairline. Hold it at 90° to the head, then cut it to the guideline from the first section. Continue down this panel to extend this guideline through the top.

(c) cutting the front   (d) cutting the centre panel

5 Take the front section forwards and hold it at 90°, then cut it to the required length for the front area. Remember: wet hair stretches, so do not cut it too short (c).

Simon Shaw

6 Return to the crown area. Take a small section, parallel to the first parting, and hold it at 90° to the head. Cut it to length, following the guideline from the first section. Continue working forward down the centre panel, always cutting to the guideline from the previous section (d).

7 Move to an adjacent panel of hair and repeat the process, making sure that the panels are connected.

8 Keep working around the top of the head, cutting the hair to the length determined by the chosen haircut shape.

9 Transfer the guideline down onto the side of the head by taking a vertical section. Continue cutting the sections through the sides to the required length. The hair length may be graduated to remove weight around the ears, if required, by angling the cut across the section.

10 As the shape develops, keep looking in the mirror to make sure that the shape is symmetrical. Consult with your client at regular intervals to confirm that the developing shape is correct, making adjustments if required.

11 Move to the crown area and transfer the guideline from the front of the first parting through to the back of the head. Take a vertical section down the central panel at the back of the head (e). Hold it at 90° to the head and cut it to the length determined by the guideline (f). Take a further section below this one. The hair length may now be graduated to remove weight in the nape by angling the cut across the section, as required.

(e) taking a vertical section at the back　　**(f) cutting to the required length**

12 Move to the adjacent panel of hair and repeat the process, as before. Make sure the panels are connected, or long hairs will be left between adjacent panels.

13 When the back is complete, move to one side of the head. If there are sideburns, note the required length and cut them to shape. Carefully outline the sideburn and the hair around the ears, then move down the sides of the nape with the tips of your scissors. Use the fingers of your other hand to guide and support the scissors or clippers whilst cutting (g).

(g) cutting the sides and sideburns　　**(h) finishing the back**

14 Repeat this on the other side of the head. Ensure that the sideburns are level (see the tip on page 36). As you create the outlines, *make sure you do not cut into the natural hairline, particularly at the sides of the nape.*

15 Dry the hair into style.

16 Return to the centre panel of hair at the back of the head (h) and finish the nape area, the neckline and the side outlines, using scissors- or clippers-over-comb techniques.

(i) cutting the neckline　　**(j) cutting the neckline square**

17 Position the client's head so that it is bent forward slightly. Carefully cut the neckline straight across to the correct height (i, j). Use the proportions of the head and neck, the length of the hair and the position of the ears to determine the length that is most suitable. The neckline may be gently tapered to create a softer effect or the corners may be rounded, if required (k).

18 Shave the areas outside the haircut outlines, if necessary (see Chapter 5).

19 Graduate the outlines to blend them with the skin, where required.

20 Finish the shape by combing, styling and dressing the hair into place (l).

Simon Shaw

(k) tapering the neckline

(l) the finished look

> **tip**
>
> ■ Remember to take into account that wet hair stretches, so do not cut it too short!

> **tip**
>
> ■ When cutting a squared neckline, the centre of the neckline should be cut slightly higher than at the sides to compensate for the skin in the centre of the neck moving further up as the head goes forward. The difference should be about 5mm. This will appear level when the head is returned to its normal position.

graduated layers

In men's hairdressing, *graduated layers* are often required on the back and sides of the haircut to produce taller, leaner shapes that are more flattering to most men.

(a) before cutting

(b) cutting the first section

Simon Shaw

1 Protect the client's clothes (a).

2 Comb the hair carefully, disentangling it where required.

3 With the hair wet, make a parting about 2cm above the hairline, going from the front to the sides, around the ears and down into the nape.

4 Comb the hair at the front of the ear down from this parting to its natural position. Lift it by the width of two fingers to create the required amount of graduation. Cut the hair to the required length (b).

5 Take another section adjacent to the first, and cut it as before (c).

> **tip**
>
> ■ When determining the correct height for the neckline you should consider the length of the neck, the position of the ears, the head shape and the length of the hair. If the neckline is too low on a short neck it will make the neck appear shorter; whilst if it is too short on a long neck it will make the neck appear longer. The best height is usually about 3–4cm below an imaginary line between the bottom of the ears, but always consider your client's wishes before cutting.

(c) cutting the second section **(d) cross-checking the back**   **(e) outlining**   **(f) outlining**

6 At the back of the ear, comb the hair forwards towards the ear, lift it the width of two fingers, and cut it to the guideline from the previous section.

7 Continue cutting the hair along this first section until you reach the nape.

8 Make the second parting above and parallel to the first. Start at the front and comb the hair to its natural fall, then lift it to the same position as before. Cut this section to the guideline created by the first section beneath.

9 Continue down the second parting, taking each section to exactly the same position where you held the hair from the first parting. Ensure that the hair is lifted by the same amount each time, or the graduation will not be consistent.

10 Make further partings, continuing up the head. Pull each section of hair to the same position and cut it to the same guideline.

11 Move to the other side and repeat the process. Ensure that the hair is pulled to the position equivalent to that on the previous side.

12 As the shape develops, keep looking in the mirror to make sure that the shape is symmetrical. Consult with your client at regular intervals to confirm that the developing shape is correct, making adjustments if required.

13 When both sides are complete, cross-check the back area to ensure that the shape is balanced and that the cut is accurate (d). This may be carried out with either scissors-over-fingers or scissors-over-comb techniques.

(g) outlining

14 When the back is complete, move to one side of the head. If there are sideburns, note the required length and cut this sideburn to shape. Carefully outline the sideburn and the hair around the ears (e, f), then move down the sides of the nape with the tips of your scissors. Use the fingers of your other hand to guide and support the scissors or clippers whilst cutting (g).

15 Repeat this on the other side of the head. Ensure that the sideburns are level (see the tip on page 36). As you create the outlines, *make sure you do not cut into the natural hairline, particularly at the sides of the nape*.

16 Dry the hair into style.

17 Return to the centre panel of hair at the back of the head and finish the nape area, the neckline and the side outlines, using scissors- or clippers-over-comb techniques. The neckline should be squared, tapered or rounded, as required.

18 Shave the areas outside the haircut outlines, if necessary (see Chapter 5).

19 Graduate the outlines to blend them with the skin, where required.

20 Finish the shape by combing, styling and dressing the hair into place (h).

(h) finished looks

the sculpture cut or 'number 1'

Different variations of the **sculpture cut** are popular with many men, but most often with young men. The name is derived from the closeness of the cut: it closely follows the features of the head, so the hair appears to be sculpted. It is also sometimes called a **number 1** after the size of the clipper comb attachment often used to achieve the cut. Longer versions of this type of cut have been called 'number 3' or 'number 4', again after the size of comb attachment used.

Traditionally this type of cut was called a **crew cut** (the length usually being equivalent to that produced with a number 4 comb attachment). However, the crew cut was often achieved with just scissors-over-comb techniques, and it required great skill to ensure the same length of cut throughout.

MK Hair Studio

channelling

MK Hair Studio

The sculpture cut produces a very masculine shape. It can be quite severe, though variations in length may be used to produce effects to suit the individual client's requirements. The looks created are very easy to manage as no blow-styling or dressing is required. Some men who are partly *bald* enjoy these looks because the shortness of the hair reduces the effect and impact of the bald areas.

The sculpture cut is particularly suitable for very *tight curly hair*, where the hair is often taken very close. Indeed, the clippers are sometimes used at the back and sides with no comb attachment, although the clipper blades are set at their longest cut. Adjustable-blade clippers are usually set to their longest setting (equal to a size 1 blade), and the detachable clippers are used with a clipper blade of size 1 or above. Lines and shapes can be **channelled** into the hair on these styles to create elaborate designs.

(a) before cutting   (b) cutting the side

(c) outlining around the ears   (d) blending the back and top

1 Protect the client's clothes.

2 Comb the hair carefully, disentangling it where required (a).

3 Start in the centre panel of hair at the back of the head. Begin cutting the hair using the clippers set to the longest setting or with a size 1 blade. Alternatively, a comb attachment can be used for a less severe effect. The best-sized comb for this look is either a number 1 or a number 2. Before you start, make sure that any comb attachment is securely attached to the clippers.

4 Place the clippers flat against the neck, just below the neckline. Using a *smooth, continuous movement*, push the clippers slowly up the head, keeping them flat against the scalp until you reach the area where you want the taper to begin: in this case the occipital bone. In a smooth *rocking* movement, *pivot* the clippers away from the head to produce the shape and length of hair that you want. Unless the top panels are to be cut this short as well, do not go higher than the occipital bone without pivoting away from the head.

5 Move to an adjacent panel of hair, and repeat the process as before. Make sure the panels are connected, or long hairs will be left between them.

6 Keep working around the head, cutting the hair to the length determined by the chosen haircut shape (b).

7 As the shape develops, keep looking in the mirror to make sure that the shape is even and symmetrical. Consult with your client at regular intervals to confirm that the developing shape is correct, making adjustments if required.

8 Move to one side of the head. If there are sideburns, note the required length for any sideburns and cut this sideburn to shape. Carefully outline the sideburn and the hair around the ears (c), then, having removed any comb attachment, move down the sides of the nape with the clippers. Use the fingers of your other hand to guide and support the clippers whilst cutting.

9 Repeat this on the other side of the head. Ensure that the sideburns are level (see the tip on page 36). As you create the outlines, *make sure you do not cut into the natural hairline.*

10 Position the client's head so that it is bent forward slightly. Carefully cut the neckline to the correct height. Use the proportions of the head and neck, the length of the hair and the position of the ears to determine the length that is most suitable.

11 The neckline must be tapered to create a natural effect, so that the hair appears to fade away. Do not cut it straight across. Use clippers-over-comb techniques and set the clippers to cut at the shortest setting, or use a size 000 blade. On longer hair, the bottom edge of the comb should be held against the skin and the clippers moved up or across the comb: the comb must be angled so that the hair will be cut shorter at the bottom and left longer towards the top. On very short hair the clippers are held directly against the scalp. Pivoting the clippers away in a smooth rocking movement blends and fades the neckline.

12 Return to the centre panel of hair at the back of the head. Using a number 1 comb attachment, or a size suitable for the length of hair required, begin to blend the hair where the top of the taper meets the hair on the

(e) cutting the top

(f) an even result, with no lines visible

(g) shaping the front hairline

crown of the head (d). Move across the head, working on small sections and ensuring that each panel is connected to the previous one, blending the two areas together to create an even, continuous effect with no lines.

13 Move across the head, following the direction of hair growth. As you cut, ensure that successive panels of hair are connected (e).

14 Blend together the top panels and the side and back panels where they meet, to create an even, continuous effect (f). You may need to remove the comb attachment to do this.

15 The front hairline may be shaped with the clippers, if required, but avoid making deep cuts into the natural hairline (g).

16 Channelling with the clippers may now be used to create lines, shapes and designs, if required.

17 Comb all the hair through, checking for any long hairs. Remove them with scissors- or clippers-over-comb or freehand cutting techniques. If possible, rinse

the hair first to remove the loose hairs and help make any longer hairs more visible.

18 Shave the areas outside the haircut outlines, if necessary (see Chapter 5).

19 Graduate the outlines to blend them with the skin, where required.

20 Finish the shape by combing the hair into place (h).

(h) the finished look

MK Hair Studio

tips

■ Always comb the hair after each movement with the clippers, to remove loose hairs and ensure that you can see clearly.

■ Remove excess hair cuttings from the client's face and neck at regular intervals, to ensure that he is comfortable.

longer layered looks

uniform layers (including razor-cutting)

In men's hairdressing **uniform layering** is not often used throughout the whole haircut, because the shape produced is too round, though it can be used to create some suitable shapes on curly hair. Uniform layering is most often used through the top of the head, with graduated layering being used at the back and sides to produce a taller, leaner and more masculine shape.

(a) before cutting   (b) sectioning at the crown

(c) cutting the central panel   (d) cutting the front section

1 Protect the client's clothes (a).

2 Comb the hair carefully, disentangling it where required.

3 With the hair wet, section the hair in two by making a parting from ear to ear across the top of the head. Take a section parallel to this parting at the crown, and hold it at 90° to the head. Cut it to length using the scissors-over-fingers technique. Make sure you cut the section straight across at 90° to the head (b).

4 Take a section going down the centre panel towards the front hairline (c). Hold this at 90° to the head and cut it to the same length. Continue down this panel, but do not cut the front section at this stage.

5 Take the front section forwards and hold it at 90° to the head. Cut it to the required length for the front (d). Remember that wet hair stretches, so do not cut it too short.

6 Return to the crown area and take a small section, again parallel to the first parting, and hold it at 90° to the head. Cut it to length following the guideline from the

first section. Continue working forward down the centre panel, always cutting to the guideline from the previous section.

7 Move to the adjacent panel of hair and repeat the process. Make sure that the panels are connected.

8 Keep working around the top of the head, cutting the hair to the length determined by the chosen haircut shape.

9 Transfer the guideline down onto the side of the head by taking a vertical section (e). Continue cutting these sections to the required length. The hair length may be graduated to remove weight around the ears, by angling the cut across the section as required (f).

(e) transferring the guideline to the sides   (f) cutting the side

10 As the shape develops, keep looking in the mirror to make sure that the shape is symmetrical. Consult with your client at regular intervals to confirm that the developing shape is correct, making adjustments if required.

(g) transferring the guideline to the back   **(h) cutting the sides**

11 Transfer the guideline from the front of the first parting at the crown area through into the back of the head (g). Take a vertical section down the central panel at the back of the head. Hold it at 90° and cut it to the length determined by the guideline. Take a further section below this one. The hair length may now be graduated to remove weight in the nape, by angling the cut across the section as required.

12 Move to the adjacent panel of hair, and repeat the process as before. Make sure the panels are connected or long hairs will be left between them.

13 When the back is complete, move to one side of the head (h). If there are sideburns, note the required length and cut this sideburn to shape. Carefully outline the sideburn and the hair around the ears, then move down the sides of the nape with the tips of your scissors. Use the fingers of your other hand to guide and support the scissors or clippers whilst cutting.

14 Repeat this on the other side of the head. Ensure that the sideburns are level (see the tip on page 36). As you create the outlines, *make sure you do not cut into the natural hairline, particularly at the sides of the nape.*

15 Cut the neckline to the shape required by the look.

16 The top layers are then cut with a razor to reduce the thickness and to create more texture and movement. The hair must be wet, so dampen it again with a water spray, if necessary. Comb the hair straight back and start in the centre panel at the front, about 3 cm back from the hairline. Do not start too near the hairline or the resulting short hairs will stick straight up! The hair is

(i) thinning with the razor   **(j) thinning with the razor**

then cut, using gentle slicing movements with the razor. The razor and comb should move down the section together as the required amount of hair is removed (i, j). Take great care, as the razor can easily cut the hair straight through.

17 Shave the areas outside the haircut outlines, if necessary (see Chapter 5).

18 Graduate the outlines to blend them with the skin, where required.

(k) applying finishing products   **(l) drying the hair**

19 Finish the shape by combing, styling and dressing the hair into place (k, l, m).

tip

■ Make sure you cut each section on the top straight across at 90° to the head or a uniform layered effect will not be achieved.

(m) finished looks

square layers

Square layers are good for creating movement and texture through the interior of a mid-length haircut. On men they are particularly suitable for longer haircuts because they produce a shape that is more square and angular, and thus more masculine. They also help make longer hair more manageable.

(a) before cutting   **(b) cutting the front**

1 Protect the client's clothes (a).

2 Comb the hair carefully, disentangling it where required.

3 With the hair wet, make a centre parting from the forehead to the nape.

4 Create two sections in the nape, running slightly diagonally from the centre parting outwards to the bottom of the ears. Starting in the middle of these two sections, comb the hair down and cut it to the required length with the scissors-over-fingers technique. Continue cutting straight across these sections to produce a square line.

5 Take two more diagonal sections, about 2 cm higher and running parallel to the first. Cut the hair to the guideline, sometimes called a baseline, which was created in the nape. Continue the baseline around onto the sides.

6 Continue working up the head, taking 2 cm sections, until all of the hair at the back has been cut to this baseline.

7 Move to the front of the head and take a diagonal section about 2 cm wide on the side from the centre parting to the top of the ears. Cut this section up from the baseline created at the bottom of the sides. Continue cutting up along the section to the required length for the hair at the front (b). Do not cut the front too short or the layers through the head will be too short.

8 Repeat this on the other side. Check that the sides are level.

9 Create a section going down the centre panel from the front hairline to the nape. Take the section at the front and hold the hair straight up at 90° to the head. Cut this to the guideline that will now be visible coming up from the sides (c). This will create a new guideline on the top that determines the length of the square layers throughout the interior of the haircut.

(c) cutting the top guideline from the sides

(d) cutting a section from the back

10 Continue cutting this guideline across the central panel to the crown area.

11 Take a next section of the central panel from below the crown area and comb it straight up to the same position as the last section on the top of the head. Cut this section to the guideline on the top to produce a square layer and retain the length at the back (d). Repeat this down the rest of the central panel, making sure that the hair is all combed straight up to the same position and cut to the top guideline.

12 Move to the adjacent panel of hair at the back and repeat the process, making sure that the panels are connected.

13 Keep working around the crown (e). Imagine that the crown is the hub of a wheel, and the panels of hair are each of the spokes. Follow this process until the hair at the back is connected with the hair at the sides.

14 If there are sideburns, note the required length and cut them to shape. Ensure that they are level (see the tip on page 36).

(e) working round the crown

15 Remove any unwanted hair from outside the outline, shaving these areas if necessary (see Chapter 5).
16 Finish the shape by combing, styling and dressing the hair into place (f).

tip

- Outlines can be achieved by cutting the hair with either close-cutting clippers or an electric razor. The outline hair may also be removed completely by shaving with a razor, which should be used following the shaving procedure described in Chapter 5, 'Shaving'.

finishing

When possible the hair should be rinsed after cutting to remove any loose hair cuttings, particularly on very short styles as the short hairs can be difficult to remove.

Styling products may then be applied, and the hair dried and dressed in accordance with the requirements of the desired look. Use the mirror regularly to check the balance and symmetry of the shape as you dress it.

Show the client the finished result and apply final finishing products if required. Provide advice and tips on after-care styling and products, as appropriate.

■ health and safety

It is important to consider health and safety when cutting hair because of the risks associated with using electricity and the risk of cutting the skin. Here are some important health and safety factors that you must consider when providing haircutting services:

avoid infection

- If the client has any cuts or abrasions on his head, or you suspect that an infection or infestation is present, you must not carry out the haircut.

- Pay special attention to hygiene when cutting hair, because of the risk of cross-infection through open cuts.

- Use only clean tools and equipment. Use alcoholic wipes and sprays to keep clippers clean and disinfected between clients.

work safely with razors

- Open and safety razors have very sharp blades and must always be handled and used with great care.

- When it is not being used or when it is being carried, always close the handle to protect the blade of an open razor.

- Never place razors or other cutting tools in your pockets.

- Always **sterilise** a fixed-blade razor before *each* use.

- When using a detachable-blade open razor, always use a new blade for *each* new client.

- Used razor blades, called **sharps**, must be disposed of correctly in accordance with your salon policy. Soiled disposable materials should be placed in sealed plastic bags for removal.

work safely with electricity

- Always handle and use electrical equipment with care, and in accordance with the manufacturers' instructions.

- Never place or use electric clippers or other electrical equipment near water.

- Do not go near electrical equipment that is lying in water – first switch off the power at the mains.

- Before commencing work, visually check that electrical equipment is safe to use. Check that the cable has not frayed or been pulled, and that the plug is not loose.

- When using and storing electrical equipment, pay attention to the position of cables.

(f) finished looks

- Never overload sockets. Do not plug too many items of electrical equipment into the same socket.

- Follow the manufacturers' instructions for the care of your scissors and clippers. To avoid damage, be sure to clean and lubricate the blades regularly.

- Electrical equipment must be regularly tested, and given a certificate of testing confirming that it is safe for use. The salon owner will ensure that this is carried out, as required.

be prepared for accidents

- Make sure that you know the whereabouts of your salon's first-aid kit.

- Keep yourself up to date with your salon's first-aid and accident procedures.

- If the client's skin is cut while you are cutting his hair, stay calm and explain what has happened. Follow your salon's first-aid and accident procedures.

   Here is an example of what you should do. Give the client a clean dressing and ask him to apply it against the cut until the bleeding stops. A new dressing or plaster may then be applied. *Do not touch the cut yourself.* If the cut is more serious, advise the client to seek medical attention as soon as possible. If any gowns or towels have been soiled, seal them in a plastic bag and launder them at a high temperature as soon as possible.

- If you cut your *own* skin while you are cutting a client's hair, stay calm and explain what has happened. Follow your salon's first-aid and accident procedures.

   Here is an example of what you should do. Excuse yourself from the client and rinse the cut under cold running water to remove any hairs. Apply a clean dressing against the cut, until the bleeding stops. A new dressing or plaster may then be applied. If the cut is more serious, seek medical attention as soon as possible. If any gowns or towels have been soiled, seal them in a plastic bag and launder them at a high temperature as soon as possible.

5 shaving

At one time shaving was one of the barber's most popular services, but the introduction of the safety razor and the electric shaver have led to its decline. More recently there has been renewed interest in shaving as a service, particularly in city centre salons that offer a full range of services to the busy professional or traveller.

This chapter looks at the techniques used for shaving and covers the following topics:

- the decline of shaving in the barber's shop
- shaving in the barber's shop today
- wet and dry shaving methods
- consultation prior to shaving
- preparation for shaving
- shaving materials – products, tools and equipment
- preparing razors for use – including setting and stropping fixed-blade razors
- beard preparation – applying hot towels and lather
- shaving techniques
- a shaving procedure
- finishing the shave
- common shaving problems
- health and safety.

■ the professional shave

the decline of shaving in the barber's shop

For over 2000 years men have visited the barber's shop regularly for shaving. Indeed, until just a few decades ago many men would visit the barber's shop *daily* for their shave.

At that time shaving was performed with an *open, fixed-blade razor*, commonly known as a *cut-throat razor*, which needed regular care to keep it in good working order. Shaving oneself with this type of razor was difficult, time-consuming and often uncomfortable. A shave in the barber's shop, however, was pleasant and relaxing: the barber would perform a *face massage*, or *facial*, as part of the service.

The introduction of the *safety razor* in about 1905 and the introduction of *electric shavers* in the 1930s made shaving at home much easier. More and more men started shaving themselves and the 'self-shaver' became a feature of modern society. Demand for the 'professional shave' declined further in the 1970s when *disposable razors* were introduced and the barber's art of shaving was in real danger of being lost.

shaving in the barber's shop today

The 'self-shaver' is not a completely new phenomenon: self-shavers have existed for hundreds of years. It is the *number* of self-shavers that has had the greatest impact on shaving as a barber's shop service.

Today most men choose to shave because it suits their personal image, or their business or hygiene requirements; shaving is an important part of their personal daily grooming routine. The barber cannot hope to change this, but he can design his services to match his client's shaving routine and experiences. Many men welcome professional advice and information on shaving, particularly if these can help them overcome common shaving problems. Shaving products, equipment and skin-care products are also in constant demand by the self-shaver. Men must still get their hair cut and for this most visit the salon. Today the opportunities clearly exist for the barber to introduce his clients to shaving services.

Here are some ideas to consider if you are interested in providing shaving services:

- Offer shaving (and face massage) services for special occasions such as weddings.
- Offer shampooing, blow-drying and shaving services to travellers and other busy men.
- Offer instruction on how to shave effectively.
- Provide advice on shaving problems. For example, many men have difficulty shaving their sideburns level – they use their ears to judge the balance, but on most people the ears are not level. You can show them how to do this correctly. You can also discuss ways of avoiding razor burn, and so on.
- Provide advice on products. It will help if you also stock these products!

shaving

The purpose of shaving is to remove the visible part of the hair and leave the skin smooth to touch. This is achieved by means of a razor or some other tool that cuts the hair close to the skin. A good shave is achieved without irritating the skin. Both men and women regularly practise shaving but here we will only consider its use on men within the salon.

The professional shave is used to remove unwanted hair from the face and neck. It may be used to outline moustaches, beards, sideburns and necklines or to remove all visible beard hair.

wet and dry shaving methods

A shave may be achieved by either wet or dry methods.

dry shaving

Dry shaving uses an **electric shaver**, which may be powered by disposable or rechargeable batteries, or by mains electricity.

There are many different types of electric shaver, but typically they all consist of a number of sharp **cutting blades** that move rapidly to cut the hair when power is applied. The blades move behind a very thin **flexible guard**, which both protects the skin and positions the hairs for optimum cutting.

Electric shavers are mostly used by the self-shaver, and are particularly suitable for the busy professional or traveller. They are easy to carry and can be used with ease in almost any location, especially if powered by batteries.

wet shaving

Wet shaving is the method of shaving traditionally used in the salon. It is achieved by means of a razor, which can either be an open ('cut-throat') razor or a safety razor.

In wet shaving the area to be shaved is prepared by the application of **lather**, **gel** or **shaving oil** prior to shaving. The hairs are then removed with a razor while they are still wet.

The open razor comprises a very sharp steel **blade** which is protected by a **hinged cover** when not in use.

Safety razors have a thin **guard** covering the blade, which both protects the skin and positions the blade and hair for optimum cutting. Several different types of safety razor are available: some are totally disposable, whilst others have a **detachable blade** that is easily replaced when a new blade is required.

consultation prior to shaving

Consultation is an essential part of any hairdressing service, and is particularly important when shaving because of the risks associated with the use of razors.

Time must always be given to discussing the client's requirements with him. It is essential that careful consideration be given to each of the following factors before any lather is applied to the face.

- What does the client want? Does he want a close shave?
- Does he have a moustache, a beard or sideburns? If so, does he wish to keep them?
- Look for signs of broken skin, abnormalities on the skin, and any unusual beard growth patterns.
- Is the beard hair coarse or fine?
- Is the beard growth dense or sparse?

> ## health and safety
>
> - A thorough consultation will ensure that you identify any adverse conditions of the hair or skin that may be present. It is particularly important to establish whether a suspected infection or infestation is present: this would prevent you from carrying out the shave. (This area is covered more fully in Chapter 2, 'Client care for men'.)

There are other factors that affect the way you carry out the shave. The following are the most important:

- hair growth patterns
- hair texture
- density of the beard
- the facial features.

hair growth patterns

Hair growth patterns are the ways in which individual hairs or a section of the beard may grow in a particular direction. Hair growth patterns must be identified, and the *'first time over' shave* should always be carried out *following* the direction of the hair growth. (Shaving *against* the hair growth at the start of the shave would cause the razor to drag, and would be very uncomfortable for the client.)

If the client requests a close shave, shaving against the direction of growth may be performed during the *'second time over' shave*. Care should be taken not to shave the hair *too* close, however, as this would irritate the skin and might cause 'ingrown hairs', particularly on men with curly hair. Ingrown hairs can become infected and may lead to conditions such as impetigo or folliculitis.

tip

■ The 'first time over' shave should always be carried out *following* the direction of hair growth.

Some clients have very strong hair growth patterns in their beard, such as **hair whorls**. In such cases, shave by following the direction of hair growth around the whorl.

tip

■ Ask your client whether there are any areas he finds difficult to shave. Each client is usually an expert when it comes to identifying problem areas on his own face!

texture

As with all hair, the **texture** of hair in a beard can be fine, medium, or coarse. *Fine hair* is easy to shave, as it creates little resistance to the razor. *Coarse hair* can be very difficult to shave and requires much more lather and massaging to soften the beard before shaving. Young men usually have fine facial hair, but as men get older their facial hair often becomes much coarser.

density

Hair **density** means the amount of hair that grows in a given area of skin. This is important to consider in shaving as the density of the growth may make it necessary to carry out a 'second time over' shave.

Young men often have sparse facial hair growth, but this becomes denser as they get older. Some men have very dense beard growth, often called 'blue beards' as the density of growth gives the skin a blue tinge which remains even after shaving. Men with very dense beards may have to shave twice a day to keep a clean-shaven appearance. Not surprisingly, they may decide to stop shaving and grow beards.

tip

■ Very dense and coarse beards should be steamed with a hot towel and well lathered before shaving: the steam and lather help to soften the beard. The lather should be massaged into the beard for a few minutes and then reapplied before commencing the shave.

preparation for shaving

the prepared client

1 Carry out your consultation with the client. Look for signs of broken skin, abnormalities on the skin, and unusual beard growth patterns.

2 Agree with your client the methods of shaving that you will use.

3 Before you begin work, gather together all the materials, products, tools and equipment you will require.

4 Position the client in a reclining chair with support for his head. Use a clean paper towel over the headrest.

5 Gown the client and place a clean towel across his chest, tucked in at the neck. Place a clean paper towel over the towel and across his shoulder (from the client's neck towards your body).

6 Your hands and nails should be clean: let your client see that you have washed them. Make sure that the razor has been prepared correctly. Show your client that you have sterilised the razor or that you are fitting a new blade – make it clear that you use high standards of hygiene in your work.

> ### tip
>
> ■ After applying lather, mark the position of any moles or dimples by removing the lather from these areas with a tissue. Always make the razor stroke moving *away* from the mole or dimple or you might cut the skin!

Simon Shaw for WAHL

facial features

To prevent damage to the skin it is important to identify and consider the client's facial features. Careful note should be made of the following:

■ the mouth

■ the width of the top lip

■ the nose

■ the shape of the jaw and chin

■ any unusual features, such as moles, dimples or scarring.

■ shaving materials, products, tools and equipment

materials

Required materials include the following. First, you will need hot and cool *towels*. Unless they are specially supplied pre-packed for shaving, these should be sterilised. You will also need a roll of *tissue paper*, for wiping used lather from the razor.

In case of any accidents, you must have access to *first-aid materials*. For small nicks or cuts you will need *styptic liquid* or *powder*. You may use a *styptic pencil*, but only once – you must use a fresh one for each new client.

To avoid the risk of cross-infection, you should wear *gloves*.

health and safety

■ Always wear gloves, to avoid the risk of cross-infection. They should be tight-fitting so that you can use the razor and tension the skin effectively during the shave.

products

To carry out the shave you will need shaving *soaps*, foam or gel, for lathering the face, or shaving oil, to ensure that the face is adequately lubricated.

American Crew

To finish you may need products such as *aftershave lotions*, *aftershave balms*, *moisturisers* and *talcum powder*.

tools

open razors

Open razors are usually used in barbering. They have either a *fixed blade*, which must be sharpened or set, or a *detachable blade*, which is disposable. Open razors, also known as 'cut-throat' razors, have a hinged handle that closes to protect the blade when not in use.

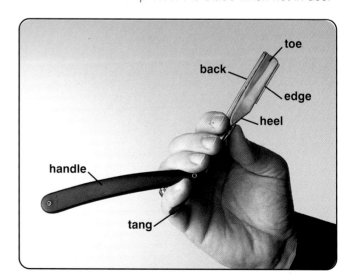

health and safety

- Open razors have very sharp blades: they must always be treated with care and respect. Keep the handle closed to cover the blade when not in use, and especially when carrying or passing the razor. Never place a razor in your pocket. Always keep razors out of the reach of children.

- When passing an open razor, the handle must always be closed. In addition, wrap your hand around it to prevent it from opening accidentally (a). Pass the razor with the tang facing away from you and towards the other person.

(a) correct: tang facing away

(b) incorrect

fixed-blade razors

Fixed-blade razors can be either 'hollow-ground' or 'solid-ground'. They were the preferred choice of traditional barbers for many years, but are more difficult to use commercially because they have to be sterilised before use on each client.

health and safety

- A different fixed-blade razor should be kept for each client's personal use: the razor should be used on no one else. Fixed-blade razors must *always* be effectively sterilised before use.

- Before using a fixed-blade razor for shaving, check your local by-laws. In many areas the use of fixed-blade razors is prohibited. (Your local council will be able to help you.)

Hollow-ground razors may be of either German or English origin. They have a concave appearance when viewed end-on, and are made of hardened steel. The steel undergoes a special heat treatment called **tempering**, which gives the razor the correct degree of hardness to produce a good cutting edge. Hollow-ground razors are usually 'hard-tempered', which makes them more difficult to sharpen (**set**), but the sharp edge lasts longer. Hollow-ground razors are light and have a particular feel that is much preferred by

a hollow-ground razor

most barbers, especially when carrying out shaving. They are less suitable for cutting hair.

Solid-ground or French razors have a wedge-shaped blade that is much heavier and more rigid than the hollow-ground razor. They too are made of hardened steel and are usually 'soft-tempered', which makes them easier to sharpen, but the sharp edge does not last as long. Due to their greater weight and rigidity they are suitable for cutting hair, but they are difficult to use when shaving.

detachable-blade razors

a detachable-blade razor

Detachable-blade razors are the preferred choice for professional shaving today because they are more hygienic than fixed-blade razors. They are designed to be very similar to a hollow-ground razor but they have

disposable blades, which are easily replaced.

The **hair shaper** is a type of detachable-blade razor that has a removable guard over the blade. These are not really suitable for shaving as the toe of the blade forms a point which can easily cut the skin when in use. However, they are good for haircutting because the guard can be left in place to help control the amount of hair being removed.

tip

Wilkinson Sword

■ Fully disposable razors may be used in the salon, but they are usually designed for home use, and are not as effective for the professional shave. Because a completely new razor is used for each client, however, they are more hygienic, and with practice they can produce an acceptable shave.

equipment

Olymp

an adjustable chair

Olymp

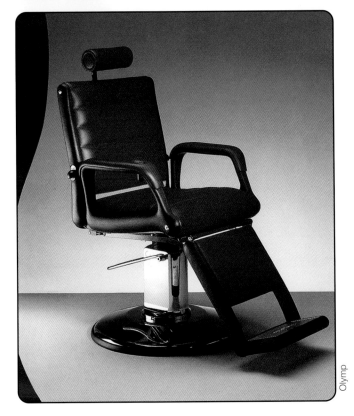

Olymp

The client should be seated in an **adjustable chair**, which can be positioned so that the client can recline comfortably while he is being shaved. It should have a **headrest**, and the height of the chair should be adjusted so that you do not have to bend uncomfortably.

A **hone** and **strop** will be required if you intend using fixed-blade razors. You may also need a **shaving brush** and a **shaving mug** or **bowl**, particularly if you intend to use shaving soaps. The shaving brush and mug must be cleaned thoroughly in disinfectant and sterilised between clients. This is often difficult to do commercially, and it is easier to keep a personal brush and mug for each client.

■ preparing razors for use

setting fixed-blade razors

Hollow-ground and solid-ground razors have to be sharpened or **set** to keep them in good working order. The process of setting a razor is commonly called **honing**, as the razor is sharpened on a hone.

Honing is a process that requires a great deal of skill to ensure that the edge of the razor is set correctly. The edge of a razor has a number of very fine teeth cut into it that have a saw-like appearance if viewed under a microscope. The teeth make the razor sharp. The process of honing sets new teeth into the edge of the razor and realigns any older teeth that remain.

The razor edge may easily be damaged or **over-honed** during honing so the razor should be tested frequently to determine the degree of sharpness. The simplest way to test the razor's edge is to place it *very carefully and lightly* on a moistened thumbnail. Slowly draw the nail along a little from the heel to the toe of the razor: if the razor tugs the nail with a smooth and steady grip, the edge is sharp.

hones

Various types of hones are available for sharpening razors. They usually consist of a rectangular block of abrasive material, which because it is harder than steel cuts the edge of the razor. Most barbers have a preferred choice of hone, acquired through years of experience.

Hones can be divided into three main groups, dependent on what they are made of: natural, synthetic, and combination.

Natural hones come from naturally occurring rock formations. They usually have to be lubricated with water or lather before use, and have a slow cutting action that produces a very fine and long-lasting edge. **Water hones**, which come from Germany, and **Belgian hones** are two popular varieties of natural hone.

Synthetic hones are man-made and can be used either wet or dry. Their cutting action is much faster than that of natural hones and they can produce a good cutting edge in less time. It is particularly important to test the razor edge regularly when using a synthetic hone, as it is very easy to over-hone a razor with a hone that cuts quickly! A **carborundum hone** is a popular type of synthetic hone.

Combination hones are the preferred choice of many barbers. They have two working sides: one side is a natural hone, the other a synthetic hone. The synthetic side is used to quickly cut a new edge on the razor. The natural side is then used to produce a very fine and long-lasting finished edge.

> ### tip
>
> ■ Great care should be taken when using a synthetic hone to avoid over-honing the razor edge.

the method of setting hollow-ground razors

1 Lubricate the hone with water, lather or oil, as recommended by the manufacturer.

2 Place the razor flat on the hone, with the edge facing towards the middle (a).

3 Using light pressure, slide the blade across the hone, moving diagonally from the heel to toe (b).

4 Rotate the razor between the thumb and forefinger whilst keeping the back of the razor on the hone – keep rotating until the razor edge is pointing straight up.

5 Using no pressure push the razor up the hone away from your body until the heel is level with the bottom edge of the hone (c).

6 Continue rotating the razor, as before, to make the blade lie flat with its edge again facing the middle of the hone (d).

7 Slide the blade back across the hone, moving diagonally from heel to toe (e, f).

8 Repeat these movements several times.

9 Every few strokes of the hone, test the development of the edge by gently and carefully placing the razor edge on a moistened thumbnail. Slowly draw the nail along a little from the heel to the toe of the razor: if the razor tugs the nail with a smooth and steady grip the edge is sharp.

stropping fixed-blade razors

The razor **strop** is used to give the razor a smooth 'whetted' edge. Stropping a razor does not cut into the steel, as honing does; instead, it cleans or polishes the

(a)   (b)

(c)   (d)

(e)   (f)

edge, depending on which side of the strop is used. There are two main types of strop available: hanging strops, and French or German strops.

Hanging strops are usually combination strops that consist of canvas on one side and leather on the other. As their name implies, they are designed to hang from a swivel attached to one end (page 81). Hanging strops are mostly used for stropping hollow-ground razors and are preferred by most barbers. **French** or **German strops** are usually made of wood and covered, again with canvas on one side and leather on the other. They are mainly used for stropping solid-ground razors and are less common.

The *canvas* side of a strop is used to clean the razor's edge and realign the cutting teeth, which become unaligned when the razor is used. The strop's effect is similar to mild honing, so a freshly honed razor should not be stropped using the canvas side. The *leather* side of a strop is made of cowhide, horsehide or imitation leather. Horsehide strops are usually of higher quality and are more expensive. The leather side polishes the edge to create a smooth finish, which is commonly called a **whetted edge**. This is achieved when all the very fine teeth on the razor edge are clean and aligned in the direction of the shaving stroke.

the method of stropping razors

The action used for stropping is similar to the action used in honing, but the razor is moved with *the back facing the direction of movement*. (Moving the razor with the edge facing the direction of movement would both cut the strop and damage the razor!)

a hanging strop

(a)   (b)

1 Place the razor flat on the strop with the back facing towards the middle (a).

2 Using light pressure, slide the blade across the strop, moving diagonally from the heel to toe (b).

3 Rotate the razor between the thumb and forefinger, keeping the back of the razor on the strop – keep rotating until the razor edge is pointing straight up (c).

4 Using no pressure, push the razor across the strop away from your body until the heel is level with the edge of the strop (d).

5 Continue rotating the razor as before, until the blade lies flat with its back again facing the middle of the strop.

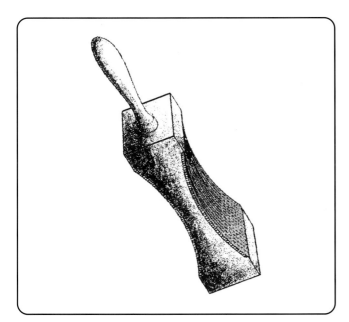

a French strop

New strops usually have to be 'broken in' before they will work effectively. Breaking in should be carried out following the manufacturer's recommendations. A method frequently used involves rubbing pumice stone across the surface to make the strop smooth. Stiff lather is then rubbed in repeatedly. Finally, and after some time, a smooth bottle or glass is rubbed over the strop until a very smooth surface is achieved.

(c)   (d)

(e)   (f)

(g)   (h)

6 Slide the blade back across the strop, moving diagonally from heel to toe (e).

7 Repeat these movements several times.

tip

■ A lot of practice is required to be able to strop a razor quickly and effectively. It is a good idea to practise with an old razor on an old strop. Make the movements slowly at first – increase the speed only when you become more proficient.

health and safety

■ Always sterilise razors after stropping.

detachable-blade razors

Used blades (known as **sharps**) must be removed carefully and disposed of in a suitable container (see 'health and safety' on page 90). The razor must then be thoroughly washed in disinfectant.

health and safety

■ A new blade must be fitted for each client.

tip

■ Show your client that you have sterilised the fixed-blade razor, or that you are fitting a new blade to a detachable-blade razor. Making it clear that you have high standards of hygiene in your work will give clients confidence.

■ preparing the beard

Ensure that the client's face and beard are visibly clean. Long beard growth that is to be removed should be disentangled as necessary, and the excess hair removed with scissors and clippers before starting the shave.

A beard must be softened before shaving is attempted. Softening the beard is achieved through the application of hot towels and lather.

applying hot towels

Hot towels steam the face and help in these ways:

- they remove dirt
- they soften the hair cuticle
- they lubricate the face, by stimulating the oil-producing glands
- they relax the muscles, making shaving easier
- they relax the client.

You must use *clean* towels. Some barbers use pre-packed towels, which are specially supplied ready-sterilised.

Hot towels are prepared in a steamer or by soaking them in hot water. Wring out the towel until it is nearly dry, then roll it up so that it retains its heat while you carry it to the client.

A towel folded ready for soaking

A rolled up towel retains heat

Unroll the towel and wrap it around the client's face, being careful not to cover the nose, so that the client can breathe. Allow the towel to cool.

The cool towel should be replaced by a second (and if necessary a third) hot towel, which should be left on while you prepare the lather.

health and safety

- Always test the temperature of the towel on the client's skin before wrapping to ensure that it is not too hot.

When using hot towels, remember the following important points:

- Always use clean towels for each new client.
- Prepare and apply the towels as quickly as possible but be sure to work safely – the quicker you are the more effective they will be.
- Avoid covering the client's nose.
- The towels should by as dry as possible when they are applied.
- Remove the last hot towel before it becomes too cold – lather should be applied to a warm face!

lathering

Effective lathering is essential to a good shave. Lathering is used:

- to remove dirt
- to soften the hair
- to lift individual hairs so that they stand erect from the skin for cutting
- to lubricate the face so that the razor glides more easily.

Traditionally the method used to produce a rich lather was to vigorously work a **shaving brush** into a bar of shaving soap and a shaving mug containing warm water. 'Working up' a good lather was necessary, as the consistency of the lather was critical to the success of the shave. The lather had to be slightly watery at first to hydrate the skin and stop the lather from drying out too quickly. The stiffness of the lather was then increased to hold the hairs erect and provide adequate lubrication for the razor.

Modern shaving products are designed to produce instant lather. They contain **conditioners** to help protect the face and to stop the lather from drying out too quickly. Some are in the form of **gels** and **oils** which do not produce lather but have the same effect. Shaving **soaps** are still available for those who wish to use them – they work well but require more preparation – so it is purely a personal choice.

Traditional lather has to be applied with a shaving brush, but modern products can be applied easily without the need for brushes or bowls. The use of the shaving brush does have additional benefits, though: the circular, upward motion used when applying the lather helps to work the lather into the beard and make the hairs stand erect.

Here are some important points to bear in mind when applying lather:

■ The lather should be applied immediately after the last hot towel has been removed.

■ The lather should be applied starting under the tip of the chin (a). It is best applied with a lathering brush in an upward, circular motion which rotates in small circles over the face (b, c).

■ The top lip is best lathered with a splayed brush, obtained by placing the index finger in the centre of the bristles (d). This avoids any lather going up the client's nose or into his mouth.

■ On dense or coarse beards, the lather should be massaged into the beard for a few minutes with three fingers of either hand, and then reapplied with the brush.

■ Do not let the lather run or drip.

(a)

(b)

(c)

tip

■ Before each shaving stroke, make sure that the lather is still creamy and moist. Dry lather will not adequately lubricate the face: this will make the razor pull, causing considerable discomfort to the client. Always apply more lather first, as required.

(d)

■ shaving techniques

The shaving procedure should be systematic. To be effective you require good co-ordination of both hands and the correct use of techniques. These are skills that take a lot of practice to develop.

You must be able to perform the techniques adequately *before* you try shaving anyone. A good way to practise is by shaving a lathered balloon with an old razor. (Ask someone to hold the balloon firmly for you while you do this.) If you burst the balloon, you were using too much pressure or holding the razor incorrectly.

This method of practising is only of use in developing 'the feel' of the razor against a delicate surface. Eventually you must make your first shaving stroke for real! You must be supervised when you do this. Work slowly and carefully, and try to remain relaxed and supple.

holding the razor

Hold the razor in either your right or left hand, as best suits you. This hand is called your **shaving hand**. The correct way of holding the razor for a right-handed person is illustrated below. For a left-handed person the razor is simply reversed.

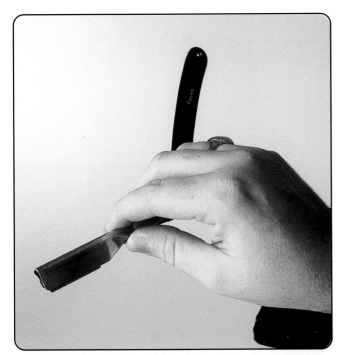

free-hand position for a right-handed person

tip

■ Try to carry out your first shave on a fine or sparse beard – this will create less resistance to the razor, be easier to achieve, and will therefore help build your confidence.

■ Avoid shaving older men during your first shaves, as older skin tends to be more 'wrinkly' and less elastic. Because it usually requires more tension to make it smooth, older skin is more difficult to shave.

back-hand position for a right-handed person

tensioning the skin

Your other hand is used to tension the skin. This is called your **tensioning hand**. You must keep the fingers of this hand dry, to prevent them from slipping on the face.

The tensioning hand should be placed at the back of the razor so that you can stretch the skin under the razor before carrying out each stroke.

shaving

The shaving stroke is performed with a single gliding movement. Try to avoid making short movements unless shaving a small area, as the razor will tend to 'pull' more and shaving will be less effective.

The free-hand stroke is made towards you, and the back-hand stroke away from you. Keep the razor at the correct cutting angle, about 40–45°, throughout the stroke. Do not apply too much pressure: the action should be light and free-moving.

Eventually you will develop a 'feel' for the correct angles and pressure to use. This feel or touch is known as the **barber's hand**, and when acquired it will allow you to make perfect shaves both safely and efficiently.

right-hand freehand stroke

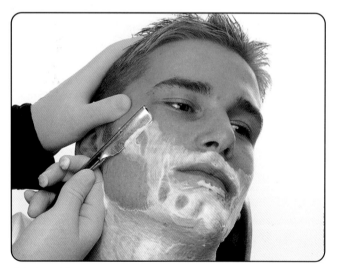

right-hand backhand stroke

■ a shaving procedure

first time over

The shave should start on the nearest side to the barber – a right-handed barber stands on the right side of the client, a left-handed barber on the left side.

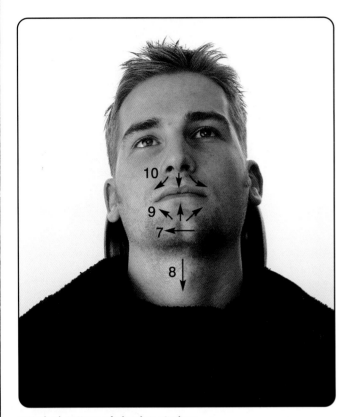

a typical pattern of shaving strokes

(a) Stroke 1

(b) Stroke 1

(c) Stroke 2

(d) Marking the sideburns

(e) Stroke 4

(f) Stroke 4

(g) Stroke 10

The skin must always be stretched taut before carrying out the stroke with the razor, otherwise cuts may occur and the shave will not be very close. After making sure they are level, mark the position of the sideburns by drawing your finger across the lather.

On the first-time-over shave, shaving follows the direction of beard growth in the pattern of ten strokes illustrated in the photographs. After each stroke, wipe the razor clean on the bottom of the tissue, then fold the tissue to cover the used lather. Keep wiping the razor this way until about three-quarters of the tissue length has been used, then replace the used tissue with a new one from the roll.

tip

- To ensure that the sideburns are shaved level, place one finger high on each sideburn. Whilst looking in the mirror slide one finger down until the desired length is reached. Slide the other finger down until both fingers are level. Mark the position of both fingers by drawing them across the lather.

health and safety

- When wiping the razor, keep the blade flat and wipe it away from the edge. Never wipe along the blade or wrap the tissue around the blade as serious cuts would surely occur.

second time over

This shave is carried out *against* the beard growth, to get a closer shave finish. This is not always required, especially on immature or fine beards.

The second-time-over shave is usually the final shave unless the client has a strong beard growth or a very close shave is required, in which case a *sponge shave* may be carried out. In the sponge shave a clean, sterilised sponge, which has been dipped in hot water, is slowly drawn across the face, closely followed by the razor. The damp sponge lubricates the face and raises the hairs into the path of the razor for close cutting. The sponge shave produces a very close shave: great care must be taken not to shave the hairs *too* close.

health and safety

- A new sponge must be used for each new client.
- Be very careful not to shave the hair too close, as this would irritate the skin and could cause ingrown hairs. This is particularly likely with curly hair.

the once-over shave

The *once-over shave* is the method used by experienced barbers to achieve a good even finish without having to re-lather the face and carry out a second time over. It is achieved by making a few more shaving strokes, as follows.

- After completing each shaving stroke, feel for remaining hair growth by running the fingers of your tensioning hand gently across the face.
- Where you feel hair growth remaining, gently complete a shaving stroke *against* the hair growth – being very careful not to shave too close.

once-over shave: shaving against the hair growth

shaving a beard outline

tip

- Extra care should be taken when shaving the outlines of sideburns and moustaches. Make sure that you mark their outline by drawing your finger through the lather before shaving. Men are often very protective of their sideburn or moustache shape, and mistakes will not go unnoticed – especially right under their noses!

the neck shave

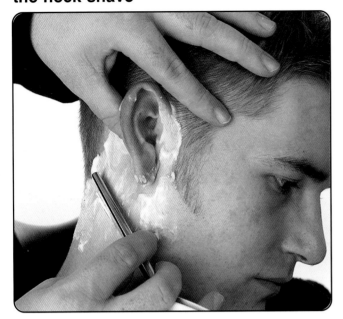

The neck shave is often used to prolong the clean appearance outside the outline of a haircut on the neck and behind the ears.

It is performed with the same techniques used when shaving the face. Note the following points.

■ The client should be gowned, with the towel placed around the back of the neck.

■ If the hair is very fine, the lather may be replaced with a little warm water.

■ Stand to the side of the client. If you are right-handed, use a free-hand stroke to shave the right side of the neck and a back-hand stroke for the left side. If you are left-handed, reverse this.

■ When shaving near the ears, protect them by folding them back gently with your tensioning hand.

■ Finish the shave by applying a small amount of talcum powder, antiseptic or moisturiser. An after-shave lotion may be applied if the client wishes.

finishing the shave

When the shave has been completed you may apply hot towels and carry out a face massage if your client requires this. If a face massage is not required, the face should be cleaned with a warm, damp towel or sponge, and then gently patted dry with a clean towel. Some clients enjoy the cooling and soothing effects of a cool

towel: this is prepared and used just like a hot towel, but using cool water. Other clients even enjoy the bracing effects of a very cold towel, but you should ask before this is applied.

American Crew

A small amount of **talcum powder** or **moisturiser** may be applied to soothe and smooth the skin. An **aftershave lotion** or **aftershave balm** may also be applied, if the client so desires. Aftershave *lotions* have a bracing effect on the skin – they are **astringent**. Aftershave *balms* are less astringent and are preferred by men who do not care for this bracing effect. Both help to close the pores of the face, reducing the risk of infection.

tip

■ Remember to comb and style the client's hair as required before he leaves the chair.

tip

■ If the client is having a face massage after shaving, apply a warm towel when the lather has been removed. The face should be warm and the facial muscles relaxed for face massage.

common wet shaving problems

The table identifies some common wet-shaving problems, possible causes and their remedies.

problem	possible cause	possible remedy
unshaven hair patches	Blunt razor Incorrect skin tension Incorrect razor angle Poor lathering	Change the blade or hone, and strop as necessary Stretch the skin smoothly before shaving Use the correct cutting angle Re-lather in the required area; re-shave uneven areas
shave not close enough	Strong beard growth Incorrect skin tension Incorrect razor angle Poor lathering	Complete a second-time-over shave and/or a sponge shave, as necessary Stretch the skin smoothly before shaving Use the correct cutting angle Apply more lather and massage in upward moves
shaving is painful	Blunt blade Shaving dry Shaving against the hair growth	Change the blade or hone, and strop as necessary Apply lather, water or oil Only shave with the hair growth on the first-time shave
shaving rash (razor burn)	Shaving dry Shaving against the hair growth Blunt razor Shaving too close Towels too hot	Apply lather, water or oil Shave with the hair growth Change the blade or hone, and strop as necessary Stop shaving Remove and cool
cuts to the skin	Blunt razor Incorrect razor angle Insufficient skin tension Too much pressure applied on razor	Change the blade or hone, and strop as necessary Use the correct cutting angle Keep the skin taut Use light shaving strokes
hair follicles inflamed	Ingrown hairs	Refer to a doctor

■ health and safety

Everyone in the salon has a duty to work safely and to keep the salon environment safe. This is particularly important when shaving because of the risk of cutting either the client's or your own skin, and the associated risk of cross-infection through open cuts. The following are some important factors that you must consider when providing shaving services.

supervision

■ Always work under expert supervision until you are competent.

consultation

■ If the client has any cuts or abrasions on his face, or if you suspect that an infection or infestation is present, you must not carry out the shave.

safety and hygiene: general

■ Use only clean towels, tools and equipment.

■ When using a fixed-blade razor, make sure it is always sterilised before each use.

■ When using a detachable-blade open razor, be sure to use a new blade for each new client.

■ Always wear tight-fitting, surgical-type gloves whilst carrying out shaves. Try not to carry out any shaves if you already have cuts or abrasions on your hands.

■ Special attention must always be given to hygiene when shaving, because of the risk of cross-infection through open cuts.

safety and hygiene: sharps

■ The use of fixed-blade razors is sometimes prohibited by local by-laws. Check the by-laws in your area before offering shaving services with this type of razor.

- Open and safety razors have very sharp blades. They must always be handled and used with great care.

- Always close the handle to protect the blade of an open razor when it is not being used or when it is being carried.

- *Never* place razors or other cutting tools in your pockets.

- Used razor blades, like all sharps, must be disposed of correctly in accordance with your salon's policy. Soiled disposable materials should be placed in sealed plastic bags for removal.

accidents and injuries

- Make sure that you know the whereabouts of your salon's first-aid kit. Keep yourself up to date with your salon's first-aid and accident procedures.

- If the client's or your own skin is nicked during shaving, the bleeding may be stopped with styptic liquids or powders. (A *new* styptic pencil may be used instead, but it must then be discarded correctly: never reuse a styptic pencil.) Any soiled gowns or towels must be sealed in a plastic bag and laundered at a high temperature as soon as possible.

- If a more serious cut occurs, follow your salon's first-aid and accident procedures.

methods of sterilisation

Sterilisation is the process of destroying *all* organisms, whether harmful or not. There are several methods of sterilisation available, which may be divided into the following groups.

moist heat

Moist heat can be applied by boiling items in **water** for at least 20 minutes, or by immersing them in **steam** and under pressure in an **autoclave**.

an autoclave

Autoclaves are the preferred choice in many salons because they are the most effective method of sterilising tools. Items in autoclaves reach very high temperatures, so make sure that the tools are heat-resistant.

health and safety

- Always take extra care when using an autoclave, and follow the manufacturer's instructions carefully.

dry heat

an oven

Dry heat is applied by placing items in an **oven** at very high temperatures. This method is most often used to sterilise sheets and towels, and is commonly used in hospitals. Some barbers use pre-packed towels which have been prepared in this way.

ultraviolet rays

Tools can be sterilised in special cabinets using **ultraviolet rays**. These are popular in many salons as they are easy to use.

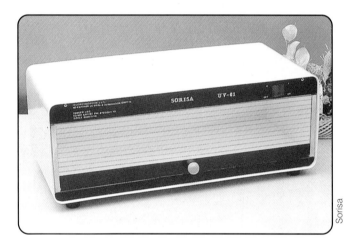

an ultraviolet-ray cabinet

All tools must be *cleaned* thoroughly before they are placed in the cabinet, as ultraviolet rays will not work effectively if the tools are dirty. The tools must also be turned regularly so that all surfaces are exposed to the rays (for about 30 minutes on each surface). Ultraviolet ray cabinets are particularly good for *keeping* clean tools sterile.

vapours

Vapours are usually formaldehyde-based. They are used in cabinets, which are also popular in many salons because they too are easy to use. As with ultraviolet rays, all the tools must be cleaned thoroughly before they are placed in the vapour cabinet, as the vapours cannot work effectively if the tools are too dirty. The tools must be turned regularly to ensure that all surfaces are exposed to the vapours for about 30 minutes. Vapour cabinets are particularly good for keeping tools sterile once they have been cleaned.

disinfectants

a disinfectant

Disinfectants are effective only if they are used in the correct strength. In the barber's shop, tools are often stored in jars of disinfectant: note that the disinfectant is no longer effective when it has become soiled. Follow the manufacturers' instructions to ensure that they are used correctly.

Many men and women enjoy the relaxing effects of a *face massage* or *facial*. At one time the face massage was a popular service in many barbers' shops, where it was often performed as part of the shaving service. The demand for face massage decreased, however, as more men started shaving at home and shaving in the barber's shop declined. More recently, though, and in common with shaving, there has been renewed interest in face massage as a service. Barbers are again offering face massage to their clients, who often request a massage at the time of their regular haircut.

This chapter looks at the traditional techniques used by barbers who provide face massage. It covers the following topics:

- face massage – the effects and benefits
- consultation for face massage
- face massage products, tools and equipment
- face massage preparation
- preparing the face for massage – applying hot towels
- face massage techniques – including effleurage, petrissage, tapotement, friction and vibro massage
- a face massage routine
- finishing the face massage
- health and safety.

tip

- Clients often enjoy having a face massage after shaving services. For weddings, some barbers offer shaving and face massage with haircutting and styling as a special service to the bridegroom and best man. Consider how you might offer these services to *your* clients.

■ face massage – effects and benefits

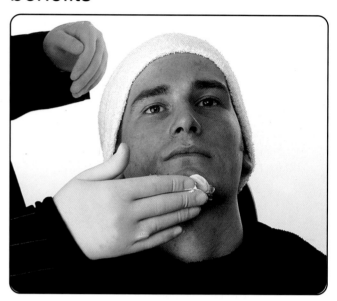

Face massage can be used to cleanse the skin and to improve its appearance, whilst providing a pleasant and enjoyable sensation for the client.

The effects and benefits of face massage include:

- cleansing and softening the skin, and removing dead epidermal skin cells
- increasing the supply of blood to the skin, to nourish the skin and to promote healthy muscles and a healthy skin colour
- stimulating and toning the underlying tissues, to help break down fatty deposits, to firm the muscles and to help define the natural contours of the face
- increasing the circulation of the lymphatic system, to help remove waste products and toxins from the skin
- stimulating or soothing of the nerves, depending on the massage technique being used
- relaxing the client, both physically and psychologically, thereby helping to relieve tension.

The massage is usually performed with the hands, which manipulate the soft tissues of the face and neck. Sometimes a mechanical massager, commonly called a *vibro massager*, is also used. A range of different massage techniques can be used to produce either stimulating or relaxing effects, depending on the client's requirements and the area to be massaged.

■ anatomy of the face and neck

For safety, anyone with an interest in providing face massage *must* understand the basic anatomy of the face and the effects that massage has on its structures and systems. It is particularly important to know the position of the **muscles** and how they act, as the massage movements should generally be performed *along* the muscle and *towards its origin*. The position of the **bones**, **nerves**, **blood supply** and **lymphatic system** must all be understood, as they affect the choice of techniques and the speed and depth of pressure with which they are applied.

bones

The bones are the foundation on which all the other structures and systems depend. The bones of particular interest in face massage are the **maxillae**, the **mandible**, the **malar** and the **nasal** bones. Other bones in the skull, known as the **bones of the cranium**, are also important in face massage, especially the **frontal**, the **sphenoid** and the **temporal bones**.

As you perform the face massage you will feel the bones beneath your fingers. In some areas of the face, such as on the forehead and around the eyes, the nose and the lips, there is little tissue between the bone and the surface of the skin. In these areas you must take care to choose the right massage technique and adjust both the speed and depth of pressure to avoid causing discomfort.

bones of the cranium

muscles

The muscles are an essential part of the face. They are interlinked with each other and with the bones to form an integrated system which allows you to eat, to speak, and to produce many different facial expressions.

Usually one end of the muscle is attached to a static bone by a strong **tendon**: this is called the muscle's **origin**. The other end is attached to a movable bone, to another muscle, or to the skin: this is called the muscle's **insertion**.

health and safety

■ If you wish to perform massage, it is important that you learn the position of muscles and their origins. Most massage movements are made along the muscle, *towards the origin* and *away from the point of insertion*. If you apply massage in the wrong places or in the wrong directions, you may cause the client discomfort.

bones of the face

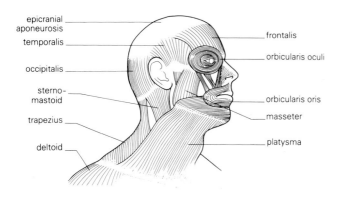

muscles of the head and face

The main muscles of the face are:

■ **occipital-frontalis** This muscle covers the top of the cranium. It enables you to lift the eyebrows, as when frowning.

■ **orbicularis oculi** These muscles surround the eyes. They help to form the eyelids and allow the eyes to close.

■ **orbicularis oris** This muscle surrounds the mouth and forms the lips. It allows you to close the mouth, and also helps in speaking.

■ **temporalis** This muscle connects the temporal bone with the malar and mandible bones. It enables you to close the mouth and helps with chewing.

■ **masseter** This muscle lies between the malar and mandible bones. It helps close the jaw during chewing.

■ **zygomaticus** This muscle goes from the malar bones to the corners of the mouth. It allows the lip to move outwards.

■ **sternomastoid** This muscle runs behind the ears to the temporal bones. It helps the head rotate and bow.

■ **platysma** This muscle, within the front of the neck, allows you to wrinkle the skin and lower the corners of the mouth.

nerves

The **nerves** carry messages to and from the brain from and to all parts of the body.

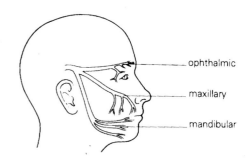

the 5th cranial (trigeminal) nerve

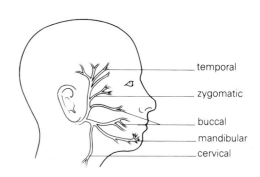

the 7th cranial (facial) nerve

In the face nerves carry messages to the skin, the muscles, the teeth, the nose and the mouth. The main nerves associated with the face are the **5th cranial nerve** (the **trigeminal nerve**) and the **7th cranial nerve** (the **facial nerve**).

Massage may be applied gently to the sites of nerve endings. During face massage, nerves may be either soothed or stimulated, depending on the technique used.

the blood supply

The heart pumps *oxygenated blood* through the *arteries* to nourish all areas of the body, including face and head. The main blood supply to the face and head is through the *carotid arteries*, which divide into smaller arteries (*arterioles*) and then into many *capillaries*.

blood supply to the head

blood vessels from the head

Eventually the capillaries join to form *venules* and then *veins*, which carry the blood back to the heart. The main veins from the face and head run down the sides of the neck, and are called the *jugular veins*.

The heart pumps the oxygen-depleted blood to the *lungs* where the oxygen is replaced. The blood then returns to the heart, and the process starts all over again.

The blood supply can be stimulated by the application of face massage techniques (see page 101).

the lymphatic system

The structure of the *lymphatic system* is similar to that of the blood supply. It is made up of a network of *lymph vessels*, *lymph nodes* and *lymph glands* which closely follow the veins throughout the body.

Its main functions are to remove bacteria, foreign matter and excess fluids from the tissues. The lymphatic system is particularly important in helping to prevent infection, and is often triggered into response when an illness strikes. You may have heard the expression 'swollen glands' – or, indeed, experienced this painful condition yourself.

lymph nodes

Lymph is a pale yellow fluid. Unlike the blood supply, the lymphatic system contains no pump. It is the movement of the larger muscles that forces lymph to move around the body. Lymph only travels away from the tissues towards the heart, not the other way.

Like the blood supply, the lymphatic system can be stimulated by the application of face massage techniques. Massage can help to promote the flow of lymph from the face and towards the lymph nodes, thereby removing waste products and toxins from the facial tissues.

consultation prior to face massage

A successful face massage will always begin with the consultation. Here you must identify your client's requirements and his reasons for wanting a face massage. It is particularly important that you assess whether the client is suitable for the massage to go ahead.

During the consultation you should discuss the client's expectations with him and provide advice on the actual results that he can expect. Take the time to explain what is involved, especially if this is the client's first face massage.

Here are some important factors that you must consider before providing a face massage:

- Make sure you establish what the client wants.

- Ask why the client wants a face massage – what are his expectations?

- Does the client have a moustache, a beard or large sideburns? Clients with long beards may not be suitable for face massage, as long beard hair is likely to pull during the massage and it is often difficult to perform the massage techniques effectively.

- Look for any signs of broken skin, abnormalities on the skin or any other *contra-indications* to carrying out the massage. Remember that the contra-indications may not always be obvious to the eye, so you should ask the client if he suffers from any skin disease or skin disorder. Make sure you do this tactfully, and take care not to embarrass the client.

- Examine the skin to determine whether its condition is normal, dry or greasy. Discuss your findings with your client and agree on the most suitable products to use.

contra-indications

Your examination of the skin will ensure that you identify any adverse conditions that may be present. It is particularly important to establish whether a suspected infection or infestation is present – if there is one, you must not carry out the face massage. (This area is covered more fully in Chapter 2, 'Client care for men'.)

Here are the most common contra-indications to face massage:

- broken or bleeding skin

- bruising, inflammation or swelling

- skin disorders, such as severe acne

- eye disorders, such as conjunctivitis

- skin diseases, such as impetigo.

Dr M. H. Beck

acne

Dr M. H. Beck

impetigo

health and safety

■ If you see any contra-indications, especially any signs of broken skin, inflammation or disease, do not go ahead with the face massage. If you are unsure, seek help from a senior colleague and tactfully advise your client to see his doctor.

■ products, tools and equipment

To provide face massage services you will need access to a range of products, tools and equipment.

products

Ellisons

Cleansing creams are available for normal, dry and oily skin types. *Massage creams* are used as the massage 'medium', to lubricate the skin and to ensure that during the massage the hands can slide easily without dragging. There are many different kinds of massage cream available: choose the correct one for your client's skin type.

Finishing products include *astringents*, which, because of their alcohol content, have a bracing and cooling effect on the skin. The cooling effect is caused by the evaporation of the alcohol from the skin. This makes the pores of the skin close and so reduces the risk of infection. *Talcum powder* may be used to ensure the skin is dry. It has a soothing and smoothing effect and can help to reduce the effect of shiny, oily skin.

tools

You will need a sterile *spatula* or *applicator* for removing the massage cream from the tub and applying it to the face.

health and safety

■ Never place your fingers directly into the tub, as this would certainly contaminate the massage cream.

equipment

You will need hot and cool *towels*, which should be sterilised if they are not specially supplied pre-packed. A *face steamer* may be used in place of the hot towels if preferred. If you wish to provide mechanical massage you will need a *vibro machine* and its applicators: some clients enjoy the intense sensation that this technique produces.

An *adjustable chair* should be available, which can be positioned so that the client can recline comfortably whilst the face massage is being carried out. If the chair does not have a *headrest* you must use some other suitable method of supporting the client's head. The height of the chair should be adjustable to avoid your having to bend uncomfortably (see pages 78–9).

◼ preparation for face massage

health and safety

◼ Always ensure that the client's head is adequately supported throughout face massage services. Check that the client is comfortable, or harm may occur!

1 Carry out your consultation with the client. Look for signs of broken skin, abnormalities on the skin and any contra-indications. Determine the condition of the skin.

2 Agree with your client the massage techniques and products that you will use.

3 Before you begin work, gather together all the materials, products, tools and equipment you will require. Place them on a trolley so that you can work efficiently.

4 Position the client in a reclining chair with support for his head, using a clean paper towel over the headrest.

5 Gown the client and place a clean towel across his chest, tucking it in at the neck.

6 Place a second towel around the head to protect the hair and keep it from falling onto the face during the massage. To apply this, first fold it in half lengthways and then in half again. Then place the folded towel around the client's head, following the hairline across the forehead. Fold the ends of the towel under and place them between the client's head and the headrest to keep the towel in place.

7 Your hands and nails should be clean. Let your client see that you have washed your hands – make it clear that you have a high standard of hygiene in your work.

health and safety

◼ Make sure your nails are not too long or they will catch the client's skin.

◼ preparing the face for massage

a prepared client

Before the massage is carried out, you must ensure that the client's skin is cleaned of any visible signs of dirt and grease. It should be cleaned using a suitable cleansing cream.

1 Select a cleansing cream to meet the requirements of the client's skin.

2 Apply the cream using a circular motion. Start at the chin and work the cream up over the cheeks, then down the jawline and neck; follow up around the lips; go over the nose and around the eyes (taking extra care); and finally across the forehead.

3 Remove the cleansing cream with clean cottonwool or tissues. Use circular strokes in an upward and outward direction. If the client has a short beard or a moustache, ensure that it too is clean. (Remember that clients with long beards may not be suitable for face massage.)

applying hot towels

The facial muscles must now be relaxed and the skin pores opened. This is usually achieved by applying hot towels; a face steamer may be used if preferred.

Hot towels steam the face. In doing so, they help:

◼ to open the pores and remove dirt

◼ to lubricate the face, by stimulating the oil-producing glands

- to increase the flow of blood to the surface and relax the muscles, which makes massaging easier

- to relax the client.

health and safety

- Always test the temperature of the towel on the client's skin before wrapping to ensure that it is not too hot.

- Be sure that the client's nose is not covered completely with the towel, as this would obstruct his airway.

You must use *clean* towels. Some barbers use pre-packed towels, which are specially supplied ready-sterilised.

Hot towels are prepared in a steamer or by soaking them in hot water. Wring out the towel until it is nearly dry, then roll it up so that it retains its heat while you carry it to the client.

Unroll the towel and wrap it around the client's face, being careful not to cover the nose, so that the client can breathe. Allow the towel to cool.

The cool towel should be replaced by a second, and if necessary a third.

When using hot towels, remember the following important points:

- Always use clean towels for each new client.

- Prepare and apply the towels as quickly as possible but be sure to work safely – the quicker you are the more effective they will be.

- Avoid covering the client's nose.

- The towels should by as dry as possible when they are applied.

- Remove the last hot towel before it becomes too cold – face massage should be performed on a warm, relaxed face!

■ face massage techniques

The face massage is performed using a variety of massage techniques, each of which produces a different effect. These techniques can be divided into two basic groups:

- manual massage

- mechanical massage

Manual massage techniques are performed with the hands and are used in virtually all face massages, and in most other massages too. *Mechanical massage* techniques require the use of a vibro machine: this imitates some of the manual massage movements, but its effect is often more intense. The vibro machine may be used on its own but is more often used in conjunction with manual massage techniques for clients who like the intense sensation that it creates.

All massage techniques should be adapted to suit the needs of the client and the area that is to be massaged. Both the *speed* of the technique and the *depth of pressure* applied may be adapted.

Remember that extra pressure should be applied only when working on the larger muscle areas.

tip

- Before you continue with a new massage movement, ask your client if the speed and pressure you are using are comfortable.

health and safety

■ Take extra care when applying massaging techniques around the eyes, nose, temples, throat and lips. Do not use tapotement or vibro techniques in these areas – the intense movement would be very uncomfortable and might cause harm. ***Never apply massage techniques directly to the eyes and ensure that you use light pressure and movements on other sensitive areas***.

manual massage

effleurage

effleurage

Effleurage is a circular, stroking movement. It is the foundation of all good massage and is used to induce relaxation, particularly at the start and the completion of the face massage. It is also used as a link between the different massage techniques, to maintain the sensation of continual massage for the client.

The depth of pressure that you apply must be adapted to take account of the thickness of the underlying tissues.

health and safety

■ The pressure should never be too deep, or discomfort and harm might occur.

The movement should be light, slow and rhythmical, so as to promote a sense of relaxation.

The main effects of effleurage are:

■ relaxation of the muscles
■ relaxation of the client
■ increased circulation of the blood supply
■ increased circulation of the lymphatic system.

petrissage

petrissage

Petrissage is performed through a mixture of *pinching*, *kneading* and *rolling* movements. It is applied with both hands, which often work together to gently lift the skin between the fingers and thumbs, where it is squeezed, rolled and pinched with a gentle but firm pressure. These movements are repeated around the fuller parts of the face in a rhythmical and systematic pattern.

The main effects of petrissage are:

■ toning of the muscles and the breakdown of fatty deposits in the tissues
■ stimulation of the sebaceous glands
■ increased circulation of the blood supply
■ increased circulation of the lymphatic system.

tapotement

tapotement

friction

Tapotement, or **percussion**, is the gentle *tapping* of the skin with the padded part of the fingertips. It is applied with both hands in a rhythmical manner to induce a pleasant and stimulating effect.

health and safety

■ Great care is needed when applying tapotement in areas with little underlying tissue, such as the forehead, eyes and lip areas.

The main effects of tapotement are:

■ stimulation of the nerves, producing an invigorating sensation

■ increased blood supply to the surface of the skin

■ toning of the muscles and the breakdown of fatty deposits in the tissues.

health and safety

■ Make sure that your fingernails are not too long before performing manual face massage, particularly when using tapotement, as long fingernails would dig into the skin.

Friction, or **vibration**, is applied to the site of the nerve endings or along the path of the nerves. It is performed by rapidly *vibrating* the fingers to produce a trembling movement, which is passed through the skin to the intended nerve.

Its main effect is:

■ stimulation of the nerves, producing an invigorating sensation.

mechanical massage

vibro massager

The *vibro massage* is a mechanical massage technique that imitates the manual massage movements of tapotement and friction.

The massage is performed with a vibrating machine, which has a range of different **applicators** for use on the scalp, face or body. A spiky applicator is provided for use on the scalp, whilst a sponge applicator and a rubber cup-shaped applicator are intended for use on the face. Other applicators may also be provided for use on the larger areas of the body.

The effect produced by a vibro massager can be much more intense than that of manual techniques, and is not enjoyed by every client.

The vibro machine can be used in conjunction with the manual massage techniques or on its own: often it is not used at all. It is operated with both hands, one directing the movements whilst the other holds the machine firmly. It is most suitable for the fleshier parts of the face.

health and safety

■ Vibro massage must *never* be used directly over delicate areas, such as around the eyes, nose, temples, throat or lips.

The main effects of vibro massage are:

■ stimulation of the nerves, producing an invigorating sensation

■ increased blood supply to the surface of the skin

■ toning of the muscles and the breakdown of fatty deposits in the tissues.

tip

■ To check that your client likes the effect of the vibro massage, first apply the technique to his arm before using it on the face.

■ a face massage routine

tip

■ The face massage should be performed *before* the client's hair has been shampooed, cut or styled, otherwise the style will be ruined during the massage.

There are several different ways of performing a face massage. The starting place, the pattern of movements and the method of completion can all be tailored to suit the client and barber. Many barbers follow a preferred routine which they have developed through experience, and use their own creativity to make the massage more pleasurable and effective. With experience you too will begin to develop your own method of working.

A good face massage will always follow these simple rules:

■ Each face massage must start and end with a relaxing massage movement, usually effleurage.

■ The sequence of massage movements should flow logically so that the sensation created is one of continuous massage. For example, do not move your hands from one area to another, such as from the chin to the forehead, without linking the movement. Use broad, sweeping effleurage movements to link these areas together.

■ Keep one or other of your hands in contact with the skin throughout the massage. Avoid any repeated stopping and starting, and try not to make jerky movements.

■ Repeat each movement several times before moving on to the next area of the face.

■ Ensure that you cover all areas of the face, unless your consultation has identified otherwise.

■ Take your time. Your goal is to make the massage pleasant and relaxing: it is impossible to do this if you rush.

health and safety

■ If the face massage follows on from a shave and the skin has been nicked during shaving, you must ensure that any bleeding has stopped before providing the face massage. Gloves should then be worn but they must be tight-fitting, surgical-type gloves or you will not be able to perform the massage techniques effectively.

a manual face massage routine

The following routine is one example of how a face massage may be performed.

1 Ensure that your client is correctly gowned and protected.

2 Clean your client's face with cleansing cream.

3 Steam the face with two hot towels.

4 Apply sufficient massage cream to lubricate the face – do not apply too much or you will overload the skin. Starting at the chin, work the cream up over the cheeks, then down the jawline and neck (a). Follow up around the lips, go over the nose and around the eyes (taking extra care), and finally go across the forehead.

(a)   (b)

5 Standing behind the client, gently lift his chin to position the head for the massage.

6 Start the massage by sliding your fingers from the client's chin up the sides of the face to the temples. Without removing your hands from the face, place the pads of the first and second fingers of each hand on the sides of the forehead. Now gently move your fingers up and down between the hairline and the eyebrows whilst moving across the forehead towards the centre (b). Use light effleurage movements to relax the client, each hand moving in alternate directions (imagine you are drawing a zigzag pattern across the forehead). Work slowly and carefully to let the client become accustomed to the sensation.

(c)   (d)

7 Move the fingers back towards the temples, then make small circular effleurage strokes up and down between the eyebrows and the hairline, working towards the centre of the forehead (c). *Repeat this series of movements at least once.*

8 Slide the fingers of both hands down the forehead to the bridge of the nose. Slide the thumbs across the bridge of the nose and cross them so that the thumb on the right hand is situated on the left side of the nose and the thumb on the left hand is situated on the right side of the nose. Using gentle pressure, slide the thumbs down and then back up the nose (d). Use slightly more pressure on the upward stroke. Take care not to depress the skin and actually block the nose. *Repeat this movement several times,* then uncross the thumbs at the top of the nose.

(e)

9 Slide your fingers down the sides of the nose and make spiralling effleurage movements across the cheeks, moving back up towards the temples (e). Slide your fingers gently under the eyes and back up to the top of the nose.

10 With each hand, place your middle finger on the eyebrow near the nose. Slide across the eyebrows towards the outer corners of the eyes. Slide down the sides of the cheeks to the corners of the mouth, and make spiralling movements back up the sides of the nose (f, g). *Repeat this series of movements at least once.*

(f)   (g)

11 Slide your fingers back down the sides of the nose to the top lip. Place the index finger of your right hand flat against the top lip: the fingertip should be level with the left corner of the mouth (h). Gently slide the finger across the top lip keeping in contact with the skin (i). When the tip of the finger reaches the right corner of the mouth, replace it with the index finger of the left hand and make the same sliding movement in the other direction (j). *Repeat this movement several times, first one hand then the other, in a gentle rhythm.*

(h)   (i)

(j)   (k)

12 Slide the fingers down to the bottom lip, and repeat the same movements there.

13 Place the fingers on the chin. Using light pinching and squeezing petrissage movements, work up along the line of the jaw to the ear lobes (k, l). Slide the fingers back down the cheeks and to the corners of the mouth; then work back up towards the top of the ear, using the pinching movements as before. Make sure you cover all of the cheeks, but *do not go too close to the eyes*.

(l)   (m)

14 Slide back down to the corners of the mouth. Using the middle fingers of each hand make two deep, rotating petrissage movements, then continue this movement up across the cheeks and to the temples. Slide back to the chin. *Repeat the movement*, but this time finishing at the ear lobes.

15 Slide your fingers back to the chin. Using your fingertips, apply a very light tapping tapotement movement and work up across the cheeks to the ear lobes and back to the corners of the mouth (m). *Repeat these movements* from the mouth up towards the temples (n, o). Develop a gentle rhythm to make the movement enjoyable.

Simon Shaw

(n)   (o)

16 Slide your fingers down the jawline back to the chin. Start on the lower lip and apply gentle rotating petrissage movements over the chin and down the neck, avoiding the Adam's apple. Cover the rest of the neck, working out from the chin (p).

(p)

17 Complete the massage routine with gentle sweeping effleurage movements under the chin, across the neck and up over the cheeks.

18 Apply hot towels to remove all traces of the massage cream. Apply cool towels, an astringent, and talcum powder if required, and dry the face (see 'Finishing the face massage', below).

> ### health and safety
>
> ■ Check that the client is comfortable at regular intervals, especially when commencing a new massage movement. Be alert to any non-verbal signs of discomfort shown by the client.

> ### tip
>
> ■ As noted, sometimes it is *necessary* to wear gloves, but you may choose to wear them at all times when you are carrying out face massage. This conforms to the highest standards of hygiene. Make sure you wear tight-fitting, surgical-type gloves or you will not be able to perform the massage techniques correctly.
> ■ A face massage should be a relaxing experience for the client: it must not be rushed. A typical face massage will take about 15–30 minutes to complete.

a vibro massage routine

The face massage may be completed with a vibro massager, used either on its own or in conjunction with the manual massage techniques. Before using it, make sure your client desires this form of massage. Confirm this by first testing the effect it produces on the client's arm.

The vibro should be used following the same pattern of movements used when applying the manual massage techniques it replaces. However, extra care must be taken, especially on bony areas like the forehead and jaw. Do not use it on the nose or around the eyes.

The rubber cup applicator is used for most face massage movements. It can produce intense, stimulating effects which some clients will not like. The sponge applicator has a more gentle and relaxing effect, and should be used after the massage cream has been removed.

> ### health and safety
>
> ■ Never use a vibro massager on the nose or around the eyes.

> ### tip
>
> ■ Little pressure is required when using a vibro massager on the face.
> ■ If the effects of a vibro massager are too strong, reduce them by placing your fingers on the client's face, and the cup on your fingers.

finishing the face massage

When the face massage is complete you should apply one or two final **hot towels** to remove all traces of the massage cream. Some clients enjoy the cooling and soothing effects of a **cool towel**: this is prepared and used just like a hot towel, but using cool water. Other clients even enjoy the bracing effects of a very cold towel, but you should ask before this is applied.

The effects of cool towels include:

■ closing the pores of the skin, thereby reducing the risk of infection

■ making the skin contract, producing a stimulating, invigorating sensation.

A small amount of **talcum powder** may be applied to soothe and smooth the skin and to reduce any shiny effect that may have appeared. An **astringent lotion** may also be applied, if the client so desires. Astringent lotions have a bracing effect on the skin: as the alcohol in them evaporates, the skin cools, closing the pores of the face, and reducing the risk of infection.

When the face massage is complete, the client's hair should be shampooed, cut (if required) and styled.

■ health and safety

Anyone providing face massage services has a duty to work safely and hygienically. You must maintain high standards of hygiene in all aspects of your work to minimise the risk of cross-infection.

The following are some important factors to consider when preparing to carry out a face massage.

check for contra-indications

■ Do not go ahead with the face massage if you see any contra-indications, especially any signs of broken skin, inflammation or disease. In these cases you should seek help from a senior colleague if necessary, and tactfully advise your client to see his doctor.

use gloves as necessary

■ If the face massage is following on from a shave and the skin has been nicked during shaving, make sure that any bleeding has stopped before providing the face massage. Wear tight-fitting, surgical-type gloves or you will not be able to perform the massage techniques effectively. Make sure you apply sufficient massage cream to lubricate the skin, as gloves can drag and pull the skin more easily.

do not harm the client!

■ Take extra care when applying massaging techniques around the *eyes*, the *nose*, the *temples*, the *throat* and the *lip* areas. **Do not use tapotement or vibro techniques in these areas**, as the intense movement will be very uncomfortable and may cause harm.

■ **Never apply massage techniques directly to the eyes**. Use only light pressure and movements on any sensitive area. Be alert to any non-verbal signs of discomfort shown by the client.

■ Keep your fingernails short. If they are too long they may catch the client's skin.

maintain a high standard of hygiene

■ Use only clean towels, tools and equipment.

■ Always pay special attention to hygiene when providing face massage: your hands will be working close to the client's mouth, eyes and nose. Always wash your hands thoroughly before you begin work, and make sure you are maintaining high standards of personal hygiene.

■ You may wish to observe the highest standard of hygiene by always wearing gloves when providing face massage services. If so, they must always be tight-fitting, surgical-type gloves.

be prepared for accidents

■ Make sure that you know the whereabouts of your salon's first-aid kit.

■ Keep yourself up to date with your salon's first-aid and accident procedures.

■ Re-read the section on methods of sterilisation in Chapter 2, 'Client care for men'.

Vidal Sassoon

Blow-drying is the art of styling wet hair with brushes, combs or fingers whilst blow-drying it with a hand-held hairdryer. Today, many men enjoy having their hair shampooed and 'blow-styled', so the barber must consider how the hair is to be professionally dried and finished.

The techniques used for blow-drying and styling men's hair are very similar to those used in women's hairdressing. Some would say there is no difference, but the barber understands that differences exist in the way that the techniques are *used*, and in the different effects that they achieve.

This chapter examines how blow-drying and styling techniques are used in men's hairdressing. It covers the following topics:

■ the theory of blow-drying

■ consultation for blow-drying

■ preparation for blow-drying

■ styling products, tools and equipment

■ blow-drying techniques – including blow-waving, finger drying, scrunch drying and natural drying

■ finishing techniques

■ health and safety.

■ the theory of blow-drying

Blow-drying works by temporarily changing the hair structure.

Wet hair is very elastic and can stretch by up to 50 per cent of its original length. It is stretchy because the weaker hydrogen bonds and salt links, which form part of the hair cortex (see page 11), are temporarily broken. The application of heat then softens the hair and causes it to stretch and mould to the new shape created by the brush, comb or fingers. The hair structure has now changed from its original state, called the **alpha state** (not stretched) to the **beta state** (stretched).

The new shape is only temporary because hair is **hygroscopic**: it absorbs moisture. Eventually moisture from the atmosphere will enter the hair and it will return to its natural alpha state. Washing the hair in hot water will return the hair to its natural state immediately.

Vidal Sassoon

■ consultation prior to blow-drying

Blow-drying is usually carried out following a shampoo or haircut, where it is used to produce the final look that the haircut has created. Consultation for blow-drying is likely to have been included in the consultation *before* the haircut, but you must still make sure that time is always set aside to discuss the client's requirements with him.

Here are some of the factors that must be considered when blow-drying men's hair.

■ Identify the client's requirements. Give him advice on suitable styles and agree the final effect to be achieved.

■ Look for signs of any unusual hair growth patterns.

■ Identify the natural fall of the hair.

■ Determine whether the hair is coarse or fine.

Many men prefer not to have too much **volume** created in the finished blow-dried style. You should pay particular attention to this during the consultation and ensure that you choose suitable brushes and techniques for creating the amount of volume required.

It may also be helpful if you read Chapter 2, 'Client care for men'.

preparation for blow-drying

Following the consultation and before you begin work, gather together all the products, tools and equipment you will require. You must also prepare the client and his hair.

preparing the client

1 Remove any wet towels and make sure your client is comfortable. If the hair has just been cut, ensure that all the hair cuttings are removed.

preparing the hair

1 Shampoo and towel-dry the hair.

2 Comb out any tangles using a comb with widely spaced teeth.

3 Apply a suitable blow-styling aid, if the hair or the style requires it. Tell your client why you advise using the styling aid and make sure your client agrees before you apply it!

products, tools and equipment

styling and finishing products

Recently, there has been a large increase in the range of styling and finishing products available that have been produced specifically for men. These products are designed to work well on different hair types and to support a wide range of style effects. They perform particularly well on short styles, which are worn by many men.

Men's products often contain little or no perfume and are available in packaging specifically designed to be attractive to men. These products work just as well on women's hair and can support many women's styles. Similarly, general styling products can be used equally well on men's hair.

American Crew

Styling products are often versatile and many can be applied to the hair either before or after blow-drying, but some products are designed for use specifically before or after blow-drying. Products that are applied *before* are designed to protect the hair and help the styling process by providing added support to the style. Products that are applied *after* blow-drying impart shine and help to achieve and retain the finished style.

Some products bond to the internal structure of the hair and help the hair to retain moisture, as well as to retain the style. Yet others are designed to help the process of moulding and shaping the hair. A good knowledge of products and their use will help you to choose the most suitable products for creating different styles and effects.

Whatever they are intended to do, most styling products will contain one or more of the following.

■ **plasticisers** These coat the hair, help mould it to shape, and then support the finished hairstyle.

■ **moisturisers** These retain the hair's natural moisture while resisting the absorption of further moisture from the atmosphere.

■ **protectors** These protect the hair from the heat of the dryer and the adverse effects of the environment, particularly from the effects of ultra-violet rays from the sun.

Two types of products are especially common in men's hairdressing today.

■ **blow-styling aids** These are used to help mould the hair into shape. They support the finished hairstyle and protect the hair from the heat of the drying process, whilst also adding volume. They are available in a variety of strengths, ranging from 'firm hold' to 'ultra hold', and they are usually available as lotions, sprays, mousses, and gels.

tip

■ Read all manufacturer's instructions carefully to ensure that you can get the best performance from their products.

■ **dressing and finishing aids** These are used to retain the finished style. Some aides can also increase the shine, and improve the apparent condition of the hair. They are often used to give definition and texture to selected sections of hair, particularly on short styles, and are commonly available as mousses, gels, creams, oils and waxes.

> ### tip
>
> ■ Manufacturers are constantly developing new styling products. Keep your product knowledge up to date by visiting the wholesalers, reading industry magazines and talking to manufacturers' representatives.

tools
brushes

Mahogany/Denman

Brushes are available in many different shapes and sizes. Next to the hairdryer they are probably the most important item you will need.

Each brush is designed for a particular purpose, although often, with experience, it is possible to achieve similar effects with different brushes. Some brushes are designed to help you dry the hair quickly and are good for general shaping. Others are good for creating volume or for creating waves.

Here are some brushes commonly used in men's hairdressing:

■ **half-round plastic brushes** These are good for creating smooth finishes and for general shaping. They can be used to build volume into the style during drying and can also be used to produce larger waves during blow-waving.

(a)

■ **half-round or straight bristle brushes** These can be either wood or plastic but in both cases they have short stiff bristles that grip the hair well (b, c). Bristle brushes are many barbers' preferred choice for blow-drying and especially blow-waving, as they can be used to produce large or small waves. They are often used to define partings and to control areas of hair without building too much volume into the style.

(b)

(c)

■ **vent brushes** Vent brushes have **vents** which allow the air to flow through easily and so aid quick drying. They are very easy to use and are often used by barbers after drying, to break up the style and create a textured effect.

■ **circular brushes** These are available in many different sizes. Small-diameter brushes are better for short to medium-length hair and produce a curled effect. Larger-diameter brushes work well on medium to long hair and produce a softer curl. Circular brushes are used more often for creating women's hairstyles than men's, but some may be used for blow-waving or for dealing with longer hair.

combs

Comby

Combs required include **wide-toothed combs** for disentangling the hair after it has been shampooed, and **cutting combs** or **straight combs** for sectioning longer hair before blow-drying. Cutting combs may also be used for creating waves during blow-waving but they must be heat-resistant.

Metal combs too are available, and are used during blow-waving. They should be used with great care, as the metal can become quite hot from the heat of the dryer. Only professional combs should be used.

tip

■ Always use a comb with widely spaced teeth for disentangling the hair or the hair will pull and may break!

equipment

Denman

The most important piece of blow-drying equipment is, of course, the **hand-held hairdryer**. There are many models to choose from, but essentially the dryer should have adjustable speeds and temperatures, and be light and easy to hold. A professional-quality dryer should be your preferred choice, as this will have several functions and be adequately constructed to give many years of trouble-free service with minimum maintenance.

Wella

The dryer must include a **nozzle** to concentrate and direct the airflow, which is particularly important for blow-waving and for men's hairdressing in general. The dryer should also have a **diffuser**, which disperses the airflow to dry the hair without moving it out of place. This method of drying produces an effect similar to that of natural drying and is often used in 'scrunch drying' (described below).

■ blow-drying techniques

Your choice of blow-drying techniques will be based upon a number of important factors:

■ the hair texture

■ the natural hair fall

■ the density (or quantity) of the hair

■ the haircut

■ the desired style.

Different types of hair may require different techniques and can produce different effects. Thick, coarse hair is often the easiest to blow-dry, as it can be moulded to produce strong effects; however, it can take longer to dry. Fine hair often requires the use of styling aids to help thicken the hair and support the finished style.

A variety of different blow-drying techniques may be used to create the different effects required in men's hairdressing. Many of these techniques are also used to dry and style women's hair, but here we will consider their use for creating men's hairstyles.

■ blow-drying

Blow-drying is drying the hair with a hand-held hairdryer. It can be used just to dry the hair, but it is usually used to dry the hair into a shape or style.

a blow-drying method

(a)   (b)

1 Towel-dry the hair and apply styling aids, as required (a).

2 Disentangle the hair, using a comb with widely spaced teeth.

3 If the hair is long, cleanly divide it into small sections, using plain clips if required. If the hair is short, use the brush to divide the area of hair you are going to dry into manageable sections. Take horizontal sections for hair that is to go down, and vertical sections for hair that is to go back.

4 Lift the section of hair with the brush, and direct the heated airflow at the root area first – but not at the scalp, or it will burn. The angle at which you lift the hair will determine the amount of volume that is created (b).

5 Work methodically and ensure that you keep any wet hair away from the hair you are drying, or have already dried. Use plain clips to secure the hair, if required. (Remember: try not to use brightly coloured clips as these might embarrass your client!)

6 During drying, always direct the airflow *away* from the roots and *towards* the ends of the hair (c). Do not direct the airflow from the ends to the roots, or the cuticles will be blown open and the hair will become dull, rough and easily tangled.

7 Keep moving the brush as you direct the warm air over the section you are drying. Visualise the moulding process that is taking place as you manipulate the dryer, brush and hair (d). Make sure the section is fully dry. If the hair is long, allow it to cool before removing your brush – or use the cold-air button on your dryer if it has one.

(c)   (d)

8 Finish the style by dressing with combs or brushes. Apply finishing products, if required.

health and safety

- Check that the temperature setting on your dryer is correct prior to starting work. Test that the temperature is suitable by directing the airflow against the back of your hand.

- Take care not to burn the hair or scalp by leaving the airflow directed in one place for too long.

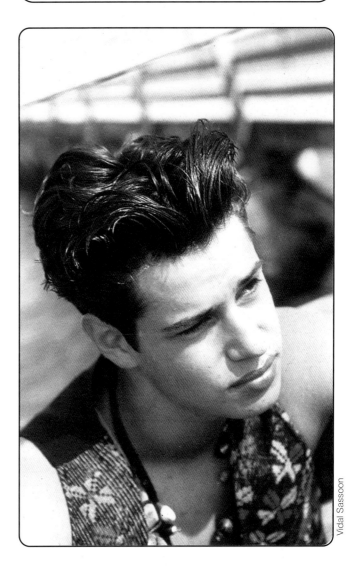

Vidal Sassoon

tip

- Many men prefer not to have too much volume created in the finished blow-dried style. Make sure you use the correct angle of lift to achieve the amount of volume required.

■ blow-waving

Vidal Sassoon

At one time blow-waving was very popular in men's hairdressing. Many men would have waves styled into their hair. Some had them going straight back; others had them going forward; yet others used waves in partings or at the sides to control the hair and keep it brushed back. Today, blow-waving is sometimes seen as being old-fashioned, and people visualise a head full of tightly formed waves. Indeed, styles full of very visible waves are not currently in vogue, but the barber understands that blow-waving skills are essential in men's hairdressing.

Blow-waving may only be used on hair that is over about 6cm in length, as the length of hair must be sufficient to allow the wave to form. It can be used very effectively to control unruly hair, particularly naturally curly or wavy hair. The waves should be created following the **natural fall** of the hair: this makes it easier to blow-wave and will ensure that the style is retained for as long as possible. It will also be much easier for clients to manage their own hair in this way.

Waves are often used *within* blow-drying to create movement that controls the hair and supports the style, in the same way that the hair may be permed to help support a desired style. The blow-drying is then completed with a vent brush, which breaks up the hair and leaves a casual finish with few or no waves visible.

tips

■ Blow-waving is much easier to achieve if you use a nozzle on the dryer.

■ Always towel-dry the hair before blow-waving, but make sure that the hair is still quite damp or the waves will not form.

health and safety

■ Take extra care not to burn the scalp when blow-waving, as the nozzle also concentrates the heat!

a blow-waving method

1 Towel-dry the hair and apply styling aids as required. The hair should be left quite damp.

2 Disentangle the hair, using a comb with widely spaced teeth.

3 Start at the front hairline and follow the hair's natural movements.

4 With a suitable brush or a wide-toothed comb, make a backward movement for about 5 cm and grip the hair. Turn the brush or comb slightly and, whilst gripping the hair, make a slight forward movement that produces the shape of a wave.

5 Direct the warm airflow along the trough created against the brush or comb, moving in the opposite direction to the brush or comb. Use a nozzle attachment on the dryer to concentrate the airflow (a).

6 Keep moving the airflow along the hair until the hair is dry, taking care not to burn the hair or scalp. Leave the hair to cool for a few seconds, or use the cold-air button on your dryer to fix the wave before moving on to the second wave (b).

7 The second wave is created in a similar way to the first, but in the opposite direction (c).

8 Keep working through the hair, creating waves where required, following the hair's natural fall. Create each wave in the opposite direction to the previous one, until the style is complete.

9 The shorter areas of hair should be dried smoothly to follow the movement of the last wave and to meet the style requirements.

10 Finish the style by dressing with a comb, or use a vent brush for a broken or textured effect (d). Apply finishing products, if required (e).

(a)   (b)

(c)   (d)

(e) the finished look

tip

■ Do not keep trying to create waves on dry hair – use a water spray and start again!

tip

■ Blow-waving is a skill that takes a lot of practice to develop. Good co-ordination is required in both hands. Practise by blow-waving just three consecutive waves before you try to do more.

contemporary blow-waving

blow-waving in contemporary styles

Blow-waving may be used to create movement that supports a wide range of styles. Many of these styles incorporate just three wave movements to achieve the required control and support.

The following method illustrates how blow-waving three consecutive wave movements may be used to produce a traditional style with a parting, without creating unwanted volume. This technique may then be applied in creating many different styles and effects.

1 Towel-dry the hair and apply styling aids as required. The hair should be left quite damp.

2 Disentangle the hair, using a comb with widely spaced teeth.

3 To find the natural parting, comb the hair back, then push it forward slightly with the palm of your hand. The hair will fall between the front hairline and the crown: this is the natural parting.

(a)   (b)

4 Start at the front hairline section of the parting.

5 With a suitable brush or wide-toothed comb, make a backward movement away from the parting for about 5 cm and grip the hair. Turn the brush or comb slightly and, whilst gripping the hair, make a slight forward movement towards the parting, to produce the shape of a wave with the trough going up towards the crown.

6 Direct the warm airflow along the trough created against the brush or comb, moving in the opposite direction to the brush or comb (a).

7 Keep moving the airflow along the hair until it is dry, taking care not to burn the hair or scalp. Do not direct the airflow too deeply into the trough. The intention is to create movement, as opposed to a full wave. Let the hair rest for a few seconds or use your cold-air button to cool the hair and fix the movement before moving on to the second wave movement.

8 The second wave movement is created in a similar way to the first, but in the opposite direction. The movement is really a series of short movements with the dryer to mould the hair around the front hairline. The trough of the wave moves towards the face. Keep working through the hair until you reach the other side (b).

9 Make the third wave movement in the opposite direction, so that the trough of the wave goes back up towards the crown (c). You will notice that this turns the hair to go down or slightly back on the side opposite the parting.

10 The shorter areas of hair should be dried smoothly to meet the style requirements.

(c)

(d) the finished look

11 Finish the style by dressing with a comb, or use a vent brush for a more broken or textured effect. Apply finishing products, if required (d).

■ other techniques

finger drying

a finger-dried look

a finger-dried look

a finger-dried look

In *finger drying* the hair is styled by pulling, teasing and lifting with the fingers while the airflow from the dryer is used to mould the hair to the shape that has been created. The method results in fullness and soft billowing shapes which have little definition and so create a casual finished look.

Justine for Charles Worthington

scrunch drying

scrunch drying

a heat lamp

Scrunch drying is used more often in women's hairdressing than men's, primarily because it is usually used on longer hair to produce a casual, ruffled effect that is particularly suitable for women. It may be used on men, but a more masculine result is often required. Scrunch drying is usually carried out with a diffuser attachment on the dryer.

natural drying

Natural drying is simply leaving the hair to dry naturally. Some men choose natural drying when it suits the hairstyle they are wearing.

In the salon, natural drying is usually assisted by the application of heat from infra-red lamps or accelerators or by blow-drying with a diffuser attachment. Essentially, the main characteristic of this method is that the hair is not styled during drying but is left to dry in its natural fall.

tip

■ When blow-drying, use the mirror regularly to check the balance of the style as it develops.

finishing techniques

After drying, the style should be finished by combing or brushing. Some styling aids may be applied at this time to help smooth the hair while it is being dressed. Use of the comb will produce a smooth result, whereas a brush is likely to produce a more broken or textured effect. Use the mirror regularly to check the balance and symmetry of the style as you dress it.

When the desired effect has been achieved, finishing aids such as hairspray or wax may be applied to help retain it.

health and safety

Everyone in the salon has a duty to work safely and keep his or her environment safe. It is important to consider health and safety in blow-drying, because of the risks associated with using electricity and the risk of burning the skin with the heat from the drying equipment.

Here are some important health and safety factors that you must consider when providing blow-drying services.

work safely with electricity

- Electrical equipment must always be handled and used with care, in accordance with the manufacturers' instructions.
- Never use or place a hand-dryer or other electrical equipment near water.
- Do not go near electrical equipment that is lying in water – switch off the mains power first.

- Before commencing work, visually check that electrical equipment is safe to use – check that the cable has not frayed or been pulled, and that the plug is not loose.
- Pay attention to the position of cables when using and storing electrical equipment.
- Never overload sockets by plugging too many items of electrical equipment into the same socket.
- Electrical equipment must be regularly tested and given a certificate of testing to confirm that it is safe to use. Your salon owner will ensure that this is carried out, as required.

avoid accidents

- Follow the manufacturer's instructions for the care of your dryer. Ensure that you clean the air filter regularly, to avoid overheating.
- Take care not to let the client's or your own hair or clothes get drawn into the air inlet at the back of the dryer.
- Always direct the airflow away from the scalp – this avoids burning, and produces a better, smoother blow-dried result.
- Use only clean tools and equipment.

be prepared for accidents

- Make sure that you know the whereabouts of your salon's first-aid kit.
- Keep yourself up to date with your salon's first-aid and accident procedures.

8 perming men's hair

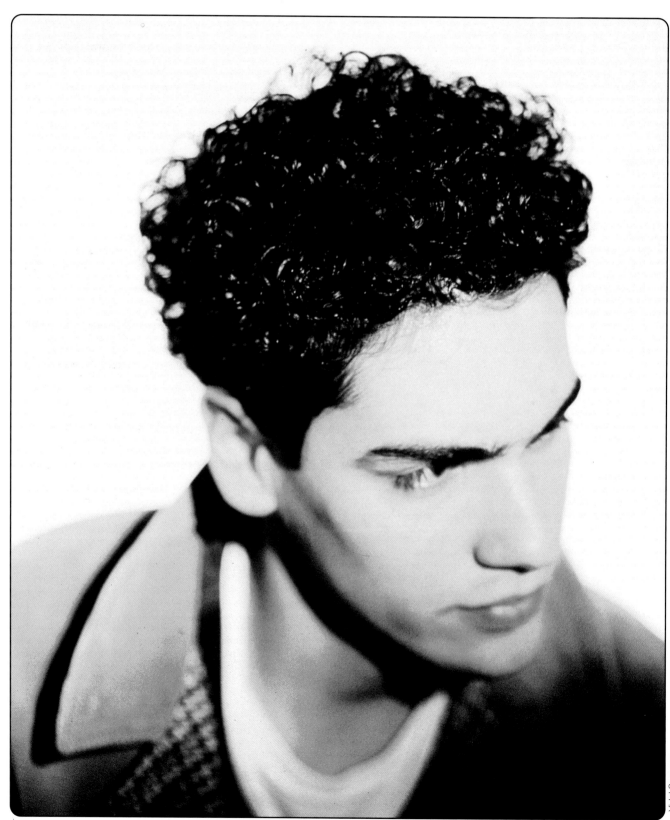

Perming is the term used to describe the physical and chemical process used to change straight hair into curls or waves. Traditionally, perming has not often been required as a service in the barber's shop, so few barbers developed or offered perming services. Perming has featured in some fashionable men's looks, such as the 'curly' looks that were popular in the 1980s, but it was mostly women who requested perming services. Today, most men still do not have their hair permed, but some men have recognised that perming can provide additional volume and control and enable them to maintain looks that would otherwise be difficult to achieve.

This chapter is designed to provide an insight into how perming can be used in men's hairdressing. If you are new to perming and intend to become expert, you will need to undertake more detailed studies of the principles and techniques of perming, which are mostly the same for both men and women. Detailed technical information on perming can be found in other books within the HTB/Macmillan series.

Here are some of the topics covered in this chapter:

- the basic principles of perming and neutralising
- consultation for perming men's hair
- perming in men's hairdressing.

perm rods, curlers and formers

■ the basic principles of perming and neutralising

Before reading this section it may be helpful if you read Chapter 2, 'Client care for men'.

Perming, also known as *permanent waving*, is a technique used to change straight hair into curly or wavy hair. It is achieved through a physical and chemical process that is applied to hair that has been wound around *formers*, such as *perming rods* or *curlers*. The shape, size and position of the formers determine the shape and size of the curls or waves that will be produced.

Permed curls and waves are permanent: unlike those produced in blow-styling, they will not straighten out when the hair absorbs water from the atmosphere. Indeed, permed curls and waves remain in the hair until they grow out, when the hair will need to be permed again if the client wishes to retain the style.

Over the years various methods have been used to permanently curl hair. The Egyptians curled hair by winding it around sticks, which were then coated in clay and baked in the sun. In the early 1900s heat was used in *hot perming* systems, but this process often left the hair dry and damaged. In the 1940s *cold perming* or *cold waving* systems were introduced. Initially these too were very harsh, but today cold perms are much kinder to the hair and cold perming is now the most popular method of perming used.

In the past, most cold perming lotions were *alkaline*. These produce good results and are particularly suitable for perming strong, coarse hair, although they may roughen the hair cuticle. Today, *acidic* perming lotions have become popular, especially for use on dry and weaker hair, because their effects tend to be more gentle.

the perming and neutralising process

The cold perming process consists of two key stages:

- reduction
- oxidation.

reduction

Most of the strength in hair comes from chemical links within it between sulphur atoms (S): these are called **disulphide bridges**. In the first stage in perming, perm lotion is used to split these, with the addition of hydrogen (H). This process is called **reduction**.

disulphide bridges

reduction involves breaking existing disulphide bridges

Following reduction, the hair is soft and pliable, and can be moulded to a new shape. The shape is determined by the rod or curler being used.

oxidation

oxidation involves forming new disulphide bridges

neutralisers

In the second stage of the perming process, the perm lotion is rinsed from the hair and a **neutralising agent** is applied, which stops the reduction. This process is called **oxidation**, **neutralising** or **normalising**. Oxygen (O) from the neutraliser combines with hydrogen in the hair, releasing water (H_2O) and forming *new* disulphide bridges. The positions of the new bridges depend on the way the hair has been moulded by the formers. When the neutraliser is rinsed away, the new bridges fix the hair in its new shape.

The most commonly used neutraliser, or **oxidant**, is **hydrogen peroxide** (H_2O_2): others include **sodium bromate** and **potassium bromate**.

---

tip

■ Always read the manufacturer's instructions carefully.

■ consultation for perming men's hair

Regis

The principles and techniques for perming men's and women's hair are mostly the same. What is different is how the techniques are used to create the effects and looks that men like.

The choice of the correct perming method, the correct lotion, and the correct processing time for each client relies on careful consideration of many different factors. Here are some of the critical factors that must be considered when perming hair.

■ Identify the client's requirements, then advise him on suitable styles, perming methods and products. Determine the types of curl or waves required to achieve the chosen style, and agree the final effect to be achieved.

■ Look carefully for signs of broken skin or any abnormalities on the skin or hair.

■ Determine whether the hair is fine, medium or coarse.

■ Consider the client's current style and haircut, particularly the hair length, together with your client's age and lifestyle.

■ If the client is a regular perming client, refer to his record card for details of previous work.

■ Determine the condition of the hair – is the hair dry, damaged or porous?

■ Carry out tests, as required.

---

health and safety

■ You must carry out a thorough consultation to ensure that you identify any adverse conditions of the hair or skin that may be present. It is particularly important to establish whether a suspected infection or infestation is present, or if the skin is inflamed, cut or grazed. If the client has any of these conditions, you must not perm the hair. (Health and safety is covered more fully in Chapter 2, 'Client care for men'.)

Remember that for any client, having a perm is a major decision: for a man it can be especially so. Always discuss your client's requirements with him and establish why he wants a perm and what he is expecting. Before starting work, make sure that perming is the correct solution for his needs. Carefully explain what is involved in perming and describe the benefits that he can expect and what after-care will be required.

TRESemmé

perming products

Wella

perming products

Here are some important things for you to cover.

■ Your client may not be familiar with the range of perms that are available, so you will need to explain their benefits and features to him.

■ Advise your client of the time perming takes and the costs that are involved. Make sure that the client agrees the course of action to be taken and that there is no misunderstanding before you commence work.

■ Make sure your client understands that perming is *permanent* – the results can last for many months!

■ Make sure that you prepare a record card for each client and accurately record all details of the service, for future reference.

■ After the perm, advise the client on how to manage the perm at home – the hair should not be shampooed for about two days and must be handled gently. Some manufacturers provide after-care information leaflets that you can give to clients.

health and safety

■ Clean all tools thoroughly after use to ensure that they are ready for the next client.

tips

■ Treat the hair gently after perming, especially when drying it into style. The perm may relax if you handle it too roughly.

■ More detailed technical information on perming for both men and women is provided in other books within the HTB/Macmillan series.

■ perming in men's hairdressing

Men are often unaware of the benefits that perming can bring, so they do not consider perming services. Perming can provide added volume and control which many men would find beneficial as it would enable looks to be achieved that would otherwise be difficult. It can also help overcome specific hair problems, such as cowlicks or double crowns.

Sometimes men are deterred from having their hair permed because the perming results they see displayed appear too feminine. At other times it is the service itself that can act as a deterrent, as some men find the perming process embarrassing, particularly if it is carried out in full view of those passing by the salon.

Here are some examples of how you can introduce men to the benefits of perming and encourage them to consider perming services where these are the best solution for their requirements.

■ Display examples of how perming can be used in men's hairdressing. Choose especially those that illustrate how perming can create masculine shapes. Use examples of such looks to support the client consultation.

■ Wherever possible, avoid using brightly coloured perming formers, capes and gowns, as these may embarrass the client.

■ Carry out perming services in areas of the salon designed for that purpose, and not in areas where other clients are only having haircutting services. Do not seat perming clients where they can be seen by passers by.

examples of men's permed looks

partial perming

Most men who have their hair permed prefer the curls or waves to appear natural. Indeed, most men's perming is carried out to produce volume and control to achieve a particular look: the permed curls or waves are barely visible when the hair has been dried and finished.

Partial perming, so called because only a section of the head is permed, is often more popular with men than *full-head perming*. Partial perming is particularly useful for clients who have long hair on the top and short hair at the back and sides, especially for styles that are dressed straight back on the top. Partial perming is also often used to provide volume or control in specific areas, though in each case the main requirement is that the permed effects appear natural.

Here are some examples of looks that may be achieved using perming.

- Perming is often best used to support the creation and maintenance of a particular look. The actual permed curls and waves are often not visible in the finished result, but they hold the blow-dried and dressed hair in place.

- Men generally want their hair to look as natural as possible, so curly perms are not often required. You need to consider the requirements of each individual client.

- Avoid producing perming results that are too round and full, as these tend to be more feminine. Remember that on most men taller, leaner shapes are more flattering.

John J. Dibbens for Staffords

Ralph Kleeli

■ health and safety

It is important to consider health and safety when perming hair because of the risks associated with using chemicals and the risk of damaging the skin. Here are some important health and safety factors that you must consider when providing perming services.

avoid infection

■ If the client has any cuts or abrasions on his head, or you suspect that an infection or infestation is present, you must not perm the hair.

■ Use only clean tools and equipment.

work safely with chemicals

■ Always handle, use and store chemicals with care, and in accordance with the manufacturers' instructions.

■ Protect your hands when using chemicals.

■ Dispose of used chemicals in accordance with the manufacturers' instructions, salon policy, and local authority regulations.

■ Check your salon's COSHH list of hazards to find out how to use products correctly.

be prepared for accidents

■ Make sure that you know the whereabouts of your salon's first-aid kit.

■ Keep yourself up to date with your salon's first-aid and accident procedures.

■ Take care not to splash the client's skin when applying and rinsing products.

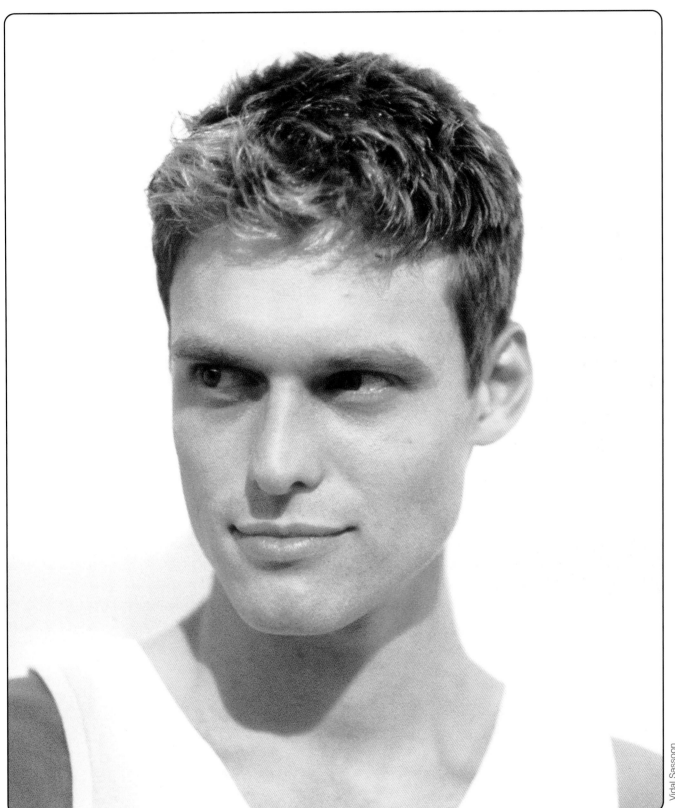

Vidal Sassoon

Traditionally, **hair colouring** has not often been required as a service in the barber's shop, so few barbers have developed or offered colouring services. Colouring has featured in some fashionable men's looks, such as the 'highlighted' looks that were popular in the 1980s. *Partial* hair colouring and **lightening** have been more popular with men: although some men have had full-head colours, usually to mask grey hairs, it has mostly been women who have requested colouring services. Today, it is still the case that few men have their hair coloured, but some have recognised that colouring can provide depth, tone and texture to enhance a new haircut or to make an old hairstyle more interesting.

This chapter is designed to provide an insight into how **hair colouring**, including **bleaching**, can be used in men's hairdressing. If you are new to colouring and bleaching and intend to become expert, you will need to undertake more detailed studies of the principles and techniques of colouring, which are mostly the same for both men and women. Detailed technical information on colouring and bleaching can be found in other books within the HTB/Macmillan series.

Here are some of the topics covered in this chapter:

■ the basic principles of colouring

■ the different types of hair colourants

■ bleaching

■ consultation for colouring men's hair

■ colouring in men's hairdressing.

■ the basic principles of colouring

Before reading this section it may be helpful if you read Chapter 2, 'Client care for men'.

some basic facts about colour

Colour helps us to interpret the world we see around us. Indeed, it is often used to provide information and instructions. Colour makes things appear more interesting and attractive. It can affect our moods, make things appear warm or cold, subdued or vibrant. On hair it can make subtle or dramatic changes to a

person's appearance, benefits that have been recognised in hairdressing for many years.

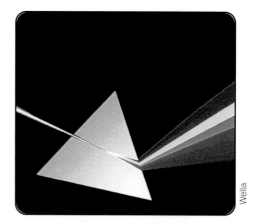

the colour spectrum from visible light

the colour circle

why we see colour

White light such as normal daylight is actually a mixture of light of many different colours. These become visible only when a prism scatters the light, or when raindrops scatters sunlight to display the different colours in a rainbow. The range of colours that we see, from red to violet, is called the visible **spectrum**.

The colours that we see are the result of different parts of the light being absorbed and reflected. Consider a red object, for example. When white light falls on this, the *red* light in the spectrum is *reflected*, and all of the *other* colours in the white light are *absorbed*. The reflected light is what reaches our eyes, so the object looks red.

natural hair colour

melanin granules in the cortex of the hair
(1μm is 1/1000th of 1mm)

colour pigments

The **natural colour** of hair is due to granules of a pigment called **melanin**. The type of this pigment, and how much there is of it, determines the colour.

Melanin is present within the **hair cortex**. The light falling on the hair passes through the hair **cuticle**, as this is **translucent**. The light is then reflected by the melanin. The colour we see is therefore determined by the colour that the melanin reflects.

There are two main types of melanin present in the hair:

■ **eumelanin** is responsible for black and brown hair

■ **pheomelanin** is responsible for red and blonde hair.

tip

■ The hair colour we see is reflected light: a portion only of the light falling on the hair. Natural daylight contains the complete spectrum – all the colours of the rainbow. Artificial lights, however, contain only some of them. Fluorescent lights tend to neutralise red and warm colours, while tungsten lights tend to add warmth and reduce ash effects. Natural daylight is the best light for showing the true hair colour.

Most people have a mixture of the two types of melanin in their hair. Their natural hair colour is formed by the quantity of each type of pigment that is present.

going grey

Age and other factors such as stress can affect the production of natural hair pigments. As we get older, our new hairs have reduced levels of pigment – or, in the case of white hair, no pigment at all.

Over time, the *proportion* of hairs on the head with reduced pigment or no pigment increases, and so the overall colour of the hair changes. **Grey hair** is the result of a large number of white hairs growing amongst the naturally coloured hairs. The amount of 'grey' hair is often described as a percentage of the whole head. For example, if half of the hairs are white and half are still naturally pigmented, the hair is described as being '50% grey'.

hair with no pigment at all

describing colour

Naturally pigmented hair colours are often simply described as being **blonde**, **red**, **brown** or **black**. Although these descriptions are adequate for general use, they are not precise enough for professional hair colouring. The **International Colour Chart** (ICC) was developed so that hair colours could be accurately identified and described – both the *natural* hair colour and the *desired* or 'target' hair colour.

Each hair colour is described in levels of depth and tone. **Depth** refers to how *light* or *dark* the colour is. This is determined by the intensity of the pigments in the hair. **Tone** refers to the *colour* that is seen. This is determined by the combination of different pigments present.

The different **shades** of colour are numbered, starting with 1 for *black* through to 10 for *lightest blonde*. Additional numbers are then added to each shade to identify the huge range of tones that are possible.

colour	depth	colour	tone
1/0	blue-black	–/0	natural
2/0	black	–/1	special ash
3/0	dark brown	–/2	cool ash
4/0	medium brown	–/3	honey gold
5/0	light brown	–/4	red/gold
6/0	dark blonde	–/5	purple
7/0	medium blonde	–/6	violet
8/0	light blonde	–/7	brunette
9/0	very light blonde	–/8	pearl ash
10/0	extra light blonde	–/9	soft ash

the International Colour Chart

▪ hair colourants

Colouring is the general term used to describe the various techniques and processes that are used to change hair colour. It is achieved through a process that adds colour pigments to the hair in the form of natural or synthetic **dyes**.

The history of hair colouring goes back many thousands of years. People have changed their natural hair colour for many reasons, sometimes to meet the requirements of a religion or society, but most often to express their individuality and create a look that they like.

colourants used

Over the years, various methods and lotions have been used to change the colour of hair. Around 2000 years ago the Egyptians used the powdered leaves of the **henna** plant to colour hair red. The Romans used a mixture consisting largely of ash, sodium bicarbonate

and lime to lighten the hair. Many other natural and artificial ingredients have been used, with varying degrees of success. In the early 1800s, however, **hydrogen peroxide** was discovered, and more modern methods of colouring were established. Today, most **hair colourants** are derived from either *vegetable* or *mineral* extracts.

colouring products

Schwarzkopf

vegetable colourants

Vegetable colourants are made from the flowers or stems of different plants, such as **henna**. For example, **camomile**, made from the flowers of the camomile plant, is used to brighten light blonde hair.

mineral colourants

Mineral colourants are made from either **metallic dyes** or **aniline derivatives**. Metallic dyes are used to coat the surface of the hair, and are sometimes used in hair colour restorers, though they are not often used in the salon.

Special care must be taken to identify whether they have been used as *metallic dyes are incompatible with hydrogen peroxide*, and peroxide forms part of many hairdressing products used in colouring, bleaching and perming. An **incompatibility test** should be carried out when the use of metallic dyes is suspected.

aniline derivatives

Aniline derivatives are synthetic dyes made from ingredients found in crude oil. They are used in most modern hair colourants and are known as **para dyes**.

These types of dye can cause a skin reaction, so a **skin test** is carried out before they are applied.

skin reaction to test

skin test for an allergic reaction

health and safety

- Follow the manufacturers' instructions for testing carefully. Do not apply products containing para dyes to a client who has had a positive reaction to a skin test. Do not apply products containing hydrogen peroxide to hair that has produced a positive reaction to an incompatibility test.

groups of colourants

Hair colourants are usually grouped according to how long they remain on the hair.

temporary colourants

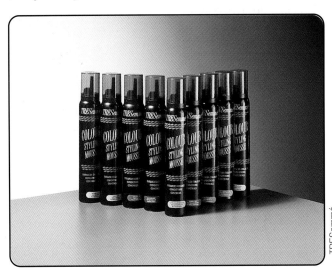

TRESemmé

temporary hair colouring products

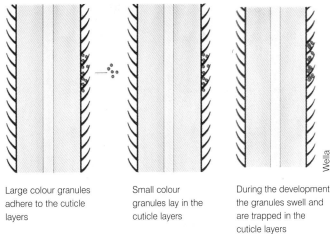

Wella

Large colour granules adhere to the cuticle layers

Small colour granules lay in the cuticle layers

During the development the granules swell and are trapped in the cuticle layers

temporary hair colouring

Temporary colourants are available as lotions, mousses, and creams, sprays gels, and so on. They contain large colour molecules which *coat* the hair cuticle. They do not penetrate into the hair cortex or affect the natural hair colour, though some temporary colours may be absorbed if the hair is very porous. Temporary colours remain on the hair until they are washed off.

semi-permanent colourants

semi-permanent hair colouring product

Large/small colour granules penetrate the cuticle layers

semi-permanent hair colouring

Semi-permanent colourants are available in several forms, though they are usually applied as a cream or rinse. Most are pre-mixed, but some have to be mixed before they are used, so it is important to read the manufacturer's instructions carefully.

Semi-permanent colourants deposit their colour molecules in the hair cuticle, and also in the outer part of the hair cortex: the molecules are smaller than those found in temporary colours. This means that the semi-permanent colour molecules are more difficult to remove, so the colour lasts longer, gradually fading as the hair is washed. The colour lasts for between six and eight washes, depending upon the condition and porosity of the hair.

Semi-permanent colourants are not suitable for covering large percentages of white hair.

quasi-permanent colourants

Quasi-permanent colourants are nearly permanent. They last longer than semi-permanent colours, but not as long as permanent colours. (The prefix 'quasi' means 'almost but not quite'.)

This type of colourant is more effective at covering white hair than are semi-permanent colourants, and it can last for up to 12 weeks.

permanent colourants

permanent hair colouring products

Permanent colourants, sometimes called *permanent tints*, are available in the form of creams and liquids, and come in a wide variety of shades and tones. They can cover white hair and naturally pigmented hair to produce natural or fashion shades, which can be very vibrant if the client so desires.

The colour molecules in permanent colourants are much smaller than those found in temporary and semi-permanent colourants: they pass easily into the hair cortex. Most permanent colourants are mixed with hydrogen peroxide. This oxidises the hair's natural pigments, causing them to combine with the molecules in the colourant and form larger molecules which become permanently trapped in the cortex.

Permanent colourants stay in the hair until the hair grows out, when the hair's natural pigmentation will again become visible. This **regrowth** must be re-coloured if the client wishes to keep his hair the desired colour.

Tiny colour granules are mixed with hydrogen peroxide – they pass through the cuticle into the cortex

Artificial depth and tone are added. Lightening of the natural pigments can occur with some shades

The granules swell and join together becoming permanently trapped

Wella

permanent hair colouring

health and safety

■ Before using permanent colourants, including toners, you must perform a **skin test**.

■ bleaching

Bleaching is the process used to make the hair colour lighter when hair colourants are not strong enough to be effective. Bleaches are available in the form of liquids, oils, creams, gels and powder.

Wella

hair bleaching/lightening product

Bleach requires a ready supply of oxygen to work. Mixing the bleach with the correct strength of hydrogen peroxide provides this. Bleach is *alkaline*. It causes the hair shaft to swell and the cuticles to lift, allowing the bleach to enter the hair cortex, where the oxygen reacts with the colour pigments, leaving them colourless.

health and safety

■ Too much bleaching will destroy the hair structure. Do not bleach hair that is in poor condition. Always avoid overlapping sections or combing bleach through hair that has been previously bleached. Before starting, process a strand of hair with a **strand test**.

tip

■ When colouring, bleaching or toning, remember to take into account the temperature of the salon. A warm room will **reduce** processing time, while a cold room will **increase** processing time.

The *eumelanin* pigment, which produces the colours black and brown, is the first to be affected; then the *pheomelanin* pigment, which gives red and yellow colours. Pheomelanin is more difficult to alter, so it becomes more noticeable as the eumelanin is lightened, sometimes making the hair appear yellow or 'brassy'. As the bleaching process proceeds, the hair gradually becomes lighter until at some point it stops getting any lighter.

The actual colour that can be achieved by bleaching depends on the proportions of eumelanin and pheomelanin in the hair. Some natural shades, such as light brown and blonde, can simply be bleached to the correct light shade. Most dark shades, however, need a **toner** applied to neutralise any remaining yellow. There are special toners made specifically for lightened hair, or diluted temporary, semi-permanent or permanent colourants may be used instead.

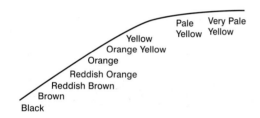

hair lightening

---

health and safety

- Take care not use too strong a solution of peroxide. Strong solutions can easily damage the hair structure and burn the skin. Avoid the bleach coming into contact with your own or your client's skin.

tip

- Always read the manufacturers' instructions and follow them carefully when using colouring and bleaching products.

bleached blonde hair

Patricia Livingston for Renbow International

■ consultation for colouring men's hair

Most of the principles and techniques for colouring are the same for both men's and women's hair. What differs in men's colouring is how the techniques are used to create the effects and looks that men like.

The choice of correct colouring method, product and processing time for each client relies on careful consideration of many different factors. Here are some of the critical factors that must be considered when colouring hair.

- Identify the client's requirements; then advise him on suitable styles, colouring methods and products.

- Look carefully for signs of broken skin or any abnormalities on the skin or hair.

- Determine whether the hair is fine, medium or coarse.

- Consider the client's current style and haircut, together with your client's age and lifestyle.

- If the client is a regular colouring client, refer to his record card for details of previous work.
- Determine the condition of the hair. Has it been previously chemically treated? Is the hair dry, damaged or porous?
- Carry out tests, as required.

---

health and safety

- You must carry out a thorough consultation to ensure that you identify any adverse conditions of the hair or skin. It is particularly important to establish whether a suspected infection or infestation is present, and to check whether the skin is inflamed, cut or grazed. If any of these conditions is present, you must not colour the hair. (This area is covered more fully in Chapter 2, 'Client care for men'.)

Remember that for any client, having one's hair coloured is a major decision. For a man it can be especially so. Always discuss your client's requirements with him and establish why he wants his hair coloured and what he is expecting. Before commencing work, determine whether temporary, semi-permanent, quasi- or permanent colouring is the correct solution for his needs.

Carefully explain what is involved in the type of colouring selected. Describe the benefits that your client can expect, and what after-care will be required. Here are some important things for you to cover:

- Your client may not be familiar with the type and range of colouring products that are available, so you will need to explain the benefits and features of each of them to him.
- Advise your client of the time colouring takes and the costs that are involved. Before you begin work, make sure that he agrees the course of action to be taken and check that there is no misunderstanding.
- Make sure your client knows how long each type of colour lasts, especially if the results will be permanent!

- Make sure that you prepare a record card for each client and note all details of the service accurately for future reference.
- After the colour, advise the client on how to manage his hair at home. The advice will differ depending upon the type of colour used. Hair that has been permanently coloured, and especially hair that has been bleached, will require careful handling and conditioning. Some manufacturers provide after-care information leaflets that you can give to clients.

---

health and safety

- Clean all tools thoroughly after use to ensure that they are ready for the next client.

---

tip

- Treat the hair gently after permanent colouring and especially after bleaching, particularly when drying it into style.

---

tip

- More detailed technical information on colouring, for both men and women, is provided in other books within the HTB/Macmillan series.

■ colouring in men's hairdressing

Men are often unaware of the benefits that colouring can bring, so they do not consider colouring services. Sometimes men are deterred from having their hair coloured because the colouring results they see displayed appear too feminine. At other times it is the service itself that acts as a deterrent, as some men find the colouring process embarrassing, particularly if it is carried out in full view of those passing by the salon.

Here are some examples of how you can introduce men to the benefits of colouring and encourage them to consider colouring services when these are the best solution for their requirements.

- Describe how colouring can provide added depth, tone and texture to enhance your client's new haircut or make his old hairstyle more interesting.

- Display examples of how colouring has been used in men's hairdressing, and especially those that illustrate how colouring can create and enhance masculine looks. Use examples of such looks to support the client consultation.

- Wherever possible, avoid using brightly coloured capes and gowns, as these may embarrass the client.

- Carry out colouring services in areas of the salon designed for that purpose, and not in areas where other clients are only having haircutting services. Do not seat colouring clients where they can be seen by passers by.

examples of colouring in men's hairdressing

Paul Stafford

Most men who have their hair coloured prefer the results to appear natural. Indeed, most men's colouring is carried out to enhance the haircut, and the colouring effects are often quite subtle. *Full head colouring* is sometimes used, but *partial hair colouring*, such as *highlights* or *lowlights*, is more popular with most men.

Charles Worthington

vibrant hair colour

A wide range of techniques and equipment may be used to partially colour hair, including wrapping hair in caps, foil or other packages, or simply applying the product onto the selected section of hair with a brush or comb.

Partial colouring is particularly useful for defining the movement and texture within a haircut, and is often preferred by clients who have longer hair on the top and short hair at the back and sides, especially for styles that are dressed straight back on the top. Colouring can also break up solid shapes and making the hair appear more disconnected and so more interesting.

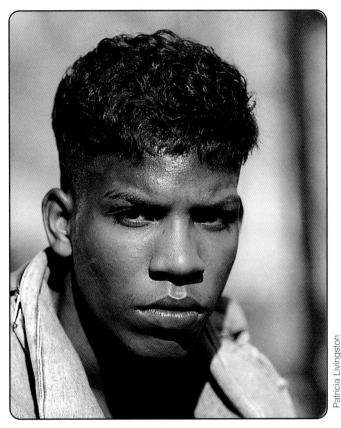

pre-lightened hair, toned with blue semi-permanent colour

Patricia Livingston

Men generally want their hair to look as natural as possible, so vibrant coloured effects are not often required. You need always to take account of the requirements of each individual client.

The following examples show how colouring can be used to enhance some common looks. In each case the colours may be lighter or darker than the client's natural base to create either highlights or lowlights. The actual choice of colour is dependent on the requirements of each client.

slicing

Slicing is good for defining movement on layered hair.

applying slices of colour to a selected section of hair

the completed application

Clynol

the finished effect

stippling

Stippling is a development of the slicing technique. It is good for enhancing textured effects in disconnected haircuts, and for defining movement.

(a) before stippling   (b) the foil in place

1 Apply barrier cream to the forehead. Place the foil on top (b).

2 Take slices across the fringe area, applying lightener as you proceed (c, d). To achieve the stippling effect, apply the lightener to a paddle brush, and brush it onto the hair (e, f). Do not overdo this, or the effects will be too solid.

(c) taking a slice   (d) the completed fringe area

3 Allow the lightener to develop, then remove it by shampooing (g).

4 Using a brush, apply the colourant to the pre-lightened hair (h, i).

5 Apply colourant to the rest of the head, straight from the bottle.

(e) applying lightener   (f) applying lightener

(g) the hair after shampooing   (h) applying colourant

(i) applying colour from the bottle   (j) the completed application

6 Allow the product to develop (j), then shampoo, condition and style the hair, as required (k).

(k) the finished effect

David Adams

3 Lightly wipe the foil across the hair, to apply colour to the ends only (d).

4 Continue applying colour over the whole of the top of the head (e).

(c) applying the first colour to the foil

(d) applying the first colour to the hair

polishing

Polishing – sometimes called ***shoeshine colour*** – is often used to create movement and texture through the ends of short layered hair.

5 Apply the second colour to the foil (f).

6 Apply the second colour, as before (g).

(a) before polishing

(b) making the hair stand up

(e) completing the application

(f) applying the second colour to the foil

1 Mist the hair lightly with hairspray, and blow-dry it to make the hair stand up (b).

2 Apply the first colour to a foil, using a brush (c).

(g) applying the second colour to the hair

7 Allow the product to develop, then shampoo, condition and style the hair, as required (h).

(h) the finished effect

David Adams

■ health and safety

It is important to consider health and safety when colouring hair because of the risks associated with using chemicals and the risk of damaging the skin. Here are some important health and safety factors that you must consider when providing colouring services.

avoid infection

■ If the client has any cuts or abrasions on his head, or you suspect that an infection or infestation is present, you must not carry out the colouring service.

■ Use only clean tools and equipment.

work safely with chemicals

■ Always handle, use and store chemicals with care, and in accordance with the manufacturers' instructions.

■ Protect your hands when using chemicals.

■ Follow the manufacturers' instructions for testing, particularly for skin testing and incompatibility testing.

■ Dispose of used chemicals in accordance with the manufacturers' instructions, salon policy, and local authority regulations.

■ Check your salon's COSHH list of hazards to find out how to use products carefully.

be prepared for accidents

■ Make sure that you know the whereabouts of your salon's first-aid kit.

■ Keep yourself up to date with your salon's first-aid and accident procedures.

■ Take care not to splash colouring products onto the client's skin or clothes, or surrounding areas.

index

Adjustable chair 79
After-care advice 9
Age 42–4
AIDS 20
Alopecia (baldness) 18, 40
Angles – in cutting 53
Aniline derivatives 132
Arrector pili muscle 15
Astringents 89, 108
Autoclaves 91

Baldness (alopecia) 40, 18
Barba 2
Barber's hand 86
Barber's itch (sycosis barbae) 16
Barber – meaning of 2, 5
Barbering – meaning of 4
Barber's pole 3
Barber surgeon 3
Beard 2, 23
Bleaching 135
Bloodletting 3
Blood supply 97
Blow drying 110, 114
Blow waving 116–19
Bones of the head and face 95
Brushes 112

Channelling 62
Children's hair 42
Client care 7
Client preparation for
  cutting facial hair 26–7
  cutting hair 47
  drying and finishing hair 111
  face massage 100
  shaving 75
Clippers 26, 45
Colour circle 130
Colour triangle 130
Colour pigments 131
Combs 46, 113
Consultation 7
Cortex of hair 11
Cuticle of hair 10
Cutting guidelines 53
Cutting techniques
  clippers-over-comb 27, 48
  club cutting 47
  clubbing over fingers 48
  freehand cutting 27, 48
  layering 52–3
  razoring 27, 49
  scissors-over-comb 27, 47
  tapering 48
  texturising 50
  thinning 50

Dandruff 18
Depth of colour 132
Dermatitis 18
Dermis 14
Diseases – bacterial viral fungal 16–17
Disinfectants 92
Drying techniques
  blow drying 110, 114
  blow waving 116–19
  finger drying 119
  natural drying 120
  scrunch drying 120

Effleurage 102
Epidermis 14
Eumelanin 131

Face
  bones of 95
  features of 25, 41
  muscles of 95
  shape of 25, 42
Face massage
  description of 94
  preparation 100
  routine 105
  techniques 101–4
Finishing
  cutting facial hair 30
  cutting hair 68
  drying hair 121
  massage 108
  shaving face 89
Fragilitas crinium 19
Friction 103
Fringes 51

Gowning and protecting 9
Grey hair 131

Hair colour – depth and tone 132
Hair colourants
  description of 132
  permanent 134
  quasi-permanent 134
  semi-permanent 134
  temporary 133
Hair dryer 114
Hair
  colouring 130
  density 25, 40, 74
  disorders 18–19
  follicle 15
  growth 13
  growth patterns 38, 74
  perming 124
  structure 10–11
  texture 24, 39, 74
  types 10, 12, 39

Hairpieces 41
Head and face shapes 25, 41–2
Head lice (pediculosis capitis) 17
Health & Safety
  colouring 142
  cutting facial hair 31
  cutting hair 68–70
  drying and finishing 121
  face massage 108
  perming 128
  shaving 90–2
Hepatitis B 20
HIV 20
Hones 79
Honing 78–80
Hydrogen peroxide 125, 132

Impetigo 16
Incompatibility test 132
Infestations 17
Insertion (muscle) 95
International Colour Chart (ICC) 131–2

Keratin 11

Lanugo hair 10
Lathering 83
Lice 17
Lifestyle 44
Lymphatic system 97

Mature men's hair 44
Medulla 11
Melanin 13, 131
Mineral colourants 132
Monilethrix 19
Moustache 23
Muscles of the head and face 95

Nasal bones 95
Neckline shapes
  rounded 37
  squared 36
  tapered 37
Nerves of the head and face 96
Neutralising 123

Once-over shave 88
Orbicularis oris muscle 96
Orbicularis oculi muscle 96
Origin (muscle) 95
Outlines 34
Oxidation 124

Partings 51
Pediculosis capitis (head lice) 17
Perming 123
Petrissage 102
Pheomelanin 131
Psoriasis 18

Razors
  detachable blade 78, 82
  disposable 78

fixed blade 77
hollow ground 77
open razors 76
preparation of 78–80
solid ground 78
Reduction 124
Ringworm (tinea capitis) 17

Salt links 11
Scabies 17
Scissors 26, 44
Sculpture cut 62
Seborrhoea 18
Sebum 15
Sharps 90–1
Shaving
  decline of 72
  description of 73
  dry shaving 73
  neck shave 88
  procedure 85–8
  shaving today 72
  wet shaving 73
Sideburns 35
Skin
  description of 13
  disorders 18–19
  structure 14
Skin test 133
Sponge shave 88
Sterilisation 91
Sternomastoid muscle 96
Stropping 80–2
Strops 80
Subcutaneous layer 15
Sweat 13
Sweat gland 15
Sycosis barbae (barber's itch) 16

Tapotement 103
Teenager's hair 43
Temporal bones 95
Temporalis 96
Tendon 95
Terminal hair 10
Tinea capitis (ringworm) 17
Tones of colour 132
Towels
  cool 89, 108
  hot 83, 100
Trichorrhexis nodosa 19

Ultraviolet rays 92
Unisex salons 5

Vapours 92
Vegetable colourants 132
Vellus hair 10
Vibro massage 104

Young men's hair 43

Zygomaticus muscle 96